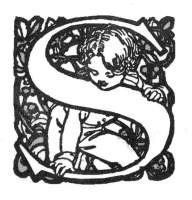

SINGLE PREGNANCY SINGLE PARENTING

Creating a Positive, Fulfilling Experience

*𝒦*ERI *ℬ*OWERS

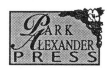

Park Alexander Press
P.O. Box 23785
Pleasant Hill, CA 94523

Library of Congress Cataloging–in–Publication Data
Bowers, Keri
Single Pregnancy – Single Parenting:
Creating a Positive, Fulfilling Experience/Keri Bowers; St. ed.
p.   cm.
Includes bibliographical references and index.

96–92334

ISBN 0–9652441–0–5

Single Pregnancy – Single Parenting books are available at special
discounts when purchased in bulk quantities for businesses, asso-
ciations, institutions or sales promotions. Please contact (toll free):

1-888-BABY AND ME
222-9263

Jacket/Book Design & Typography, Floyd P. Busby
Cover Photograph, Allison Cane
Edited by Laurel Airica

Printed in the United States of America

This book is not intended to replace the advice of legal, medical and/or mental health professionals. The information contained
in this book is intended to provide ideas, guidance, and support in
your journey through single pregnancy and parenting. The author
urges you to consult with medical, legal, psychological and other
professionals concerning questions or problems which you may encounter along the way.

The author has made every possible effort to make this book as
complete and accurate as possible. Any errors as to content in this
book are purely accidental and thus the text should be used only as a
guide and not as the ultimate source of information for the issues
related to pregnancy and parenting. The publisher and author takes
no responsibility for errors or omissions.

To Taylor and Jace —
for teaching me love and
giving me wings upon which to fly.

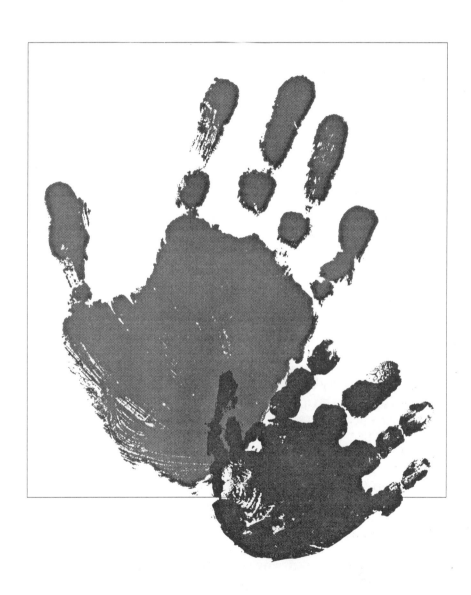

CONTENTS

CHAPTER FOUR
TAKING CARE OF YOUR BODY

CHAPTER FIVE
YOUR MOODS AND FEELINGS

CHAPTER SIX
YOUR MIND AND SPIRIT

CHAPTER ELEVEN
YOUR CHILD'S DEVELOPMENT

CHAPTER TWELVE
YOUR BABY'S FATHER

CHAPTER THIRTEEN
MORE LEGAL ISSUES

$\mathscr{A}$CKNOWLEDGEMENTS

Much like a newborn child, Single Pregnancy – Single Parenting started out, at its conception, as a seed. Then it developed a viable life of its own — eager to come into the world to share its many gifts.

Along the way, the expertise, assistance and loving acts of professionals and friends alike were generously given to encourage and sustain its life. For all of those people, I am indebted and truly thankful.

My heartfelt thanks and love go to Valerie, who gave me the foundation to aspire to greater heights — and for giving me strength when I was on empty. To Deborah, my life's blood and sustenance, there are not enough words to express my love for you.

To Jordana, Roman, Julie, Danny Jr., and Kristen — I couldn't love you more if you were my own children. To Danny — though you gave me hell — you gave me a beautiful child. I am eternally grateful. And to Ken -- though you may never understand — I owe you thanks and appreciation.

To my mother, I simply say, I love you.

To my special friends, Stephanie D., Stephanie G., Mary, Alison, Karen, Kathleen, Gail, Pamela, David, Sharri, Tim, Kelly, Delia, and Rima, thank you for all the feedback, encouragement and love you so freely gave.

A special thanks to Michael for your continued support and encouragement each step of the way. And to Amanda — thank you for all the hours you watched my boys so I could write. You are truly appreciated.

To Laurel, Scott, and Floyd, Robert, Bob, Melissa, Stephan Patricia, Paula, and Jonathan — thank you for your efforts and talents.

To all the women who gave their time to talk with me — though you are too numerous to thank individually — I am indebted to each of you. Your stories were truly inspirational. And to all my little artists with love and appreciation..

A dedication of love and rememberance to Erin. You gave me more than you know. Your legacy of love will forever be with Ryan.

And finally, to the children of single mothers everywhere — God bless you.

The DOCTOR'S, THERAPIST'S AND LAWYER'S PAGES

FROM THE DOCTOR

SINGLE PREGNANCY – SINGLE PARENTING is an upbeat and unromanticized guide to the joys and challenges of single pregnancy and parenthood, filled with down–to– earth advice, solid medical information and excellent resources.

Dr. Paula Bernstein, Ph.D., M.D.
Beverly Hills, California

FROM THE THERAPIST

While reading Keri Bowers' book, SINGLE PREGNANCY – SINGLE PARENTING, I was struck by how inspiring and supportive she is toward single parents. Psychologically, this is very critical when women, especially young women, transition into parenthood. Women need to feel confident in handling daily work, social and family obligations before they can incorporate the added responsibilities of child rearing. Keri understands that single parents have special needs that have not been fully recognized by our society.

A new child needs protection and nurturing so she can productively transition through the development stages imperative for emotional and physical growth. Too often parents are not capable of promoting proper attachment, identity and intimacy stages of development. SINGLE PREGNANCY – SINGLE PARENTING is so effective because it supports and presents a balanced "whole person perspective". Critical ingredients to self esteem include emotional, social, physical, intellectual and spiritual areas. Keri helps single women by educating them for the need to maintain this healthy balance throughout pregnancy. She sets up conditions necessary to produce children who are at less risk for wounding in their early and formative stages of development.

In addition to the single pregnant women and mothers it speaks to, I would recommend any social worker, therapist, or teacher working with women to read this book and to offer it as a resource, even before pregnancy. This book definitely helps to prepare women for the huge leap from being single to single and parenting.

Melissa Roccio, MFCC
Los Angeles, California

FROM THE LAWYER

These last few decades have established women as an integral part of our society's work force at every level of employment and career path. While today's woman continued her growth and success as a career person, the notion of traditional family of husband and wife, with wife as homemaker, has been literally cast aside for career opportunities as well as financial necessity. Moreover, with much greater demand on time and much less willingness to settle for a husband without all the qualities now demanded for a lifetime partner, it is no wonder that today's woman has such a hard time finding Mr. Right. Nonetheless, there is still the yearning to have children without a significant other. There of course remains the ever–growing phenomenon of unplanned pregnancies between unmarried individuals, adults and ever–increasingly, minors alike.

SINGLE PREGNANCY – SINGLE PARENTING provides powerful insight and resources to any woman going through pregnancy, childbirth, and the raising of a child without the help, support and companionship of such a significant other. I would recommend this book to everyone facing the fears, challenges, goals, and ultimate rewards of having and raising children as a single parent.

Jonathan A. Zahler,
Family Law Attorney,
Jacksonville, Florida

*I*NTRODUCTION

Character cannot be developed in ease and quiet.
Only through experience of trial and suffering
can the soul be strengthened, vision cleared,
ambition inspired and success achieved.

Helen Keller

According to the National Center for Health Statistics, since 1960, births to unmarried women have increased by approximately 400 percent. In 1960, 5.3 percent of all births were out–of–wedlock, and by 1994, 26 percent of all births were out–of–wedlock. In simple numbers, this means that today one child in four is born to a single mother. Clearly, out–of–wedlock births are a phenomenon that society, and single mothers, must address in order to meet the needs of children who grow up without fathers in an era of unprecedented challenge and change.

Women become single mothers through a variety of circumstances, including divorce; separation; the death of their spouse; deliberate choice; and accidental conception. Yet despite the size of the phenomenon, and its direct impact on society, little has been written to help these women deal with the particular stresses on their lives as they shape a significant portion of our next generation on their own.

I am the single mother of two young sons. You will find my story at the end of this book. While I never intended to have children by myself, the experience has been transforming and rewarding beyond what I could have foreseen; and now I would not trade my life with anyone.

I have written this book for my "sisters" — and all who assist them – – to shed some light on the many issues and emotions that must be faced and dealt with in order to create optimal child–bearing and child–rearing experiences for single mothers and their children.

I will not sugar–coat or glamorize the realities, difficulties, or far–reaching implications of solo parenting. But I will take every opportunity to point out that each of us has the power within us to make the best of every moment; and to create positive, loving and fulfilling relationships with our children, regardless of our situation.

As a single mother, your particular set of circumstances may be more difficult than you ever could have imagined. Yet even so, your problems are not insurmountable. As you are willing (and able) to embrace and use the concepts set forth in the coming chapters, and learn to make responsible choices; you will see that you have the ability to improve the conditions of your life, no matter what they are.

The key to this power is awareness and intention. The more willing you are to accept responsibility for your life — and the more conscious you are of the choices you have — the better able you will be to make mature decisions. With this as your intention, even adversity can become an ally, continually prodding you to grow beyond any limited belief in your own potential.

Within the pages of this book, you will find practical suggestions, tools, and exercises that can enhance your experience throughout pregnancy and early motherhood. However, they do not guarantee that you will not have feelings of loss, confusion, sadness, fear, anger, resentment, loneliness, etc. — because such feelings are a part of life. But they will help you learn how to gain the most from everything you encounter.

In addition to offering you tools to do the work that is before you; this "blueprint" is intended to serve as a subtle — and sometimes not–so–subtle reminder — that when you experience pain, conflict or crisis it is your responsibility to take action to change the situation. Single parenting is not a path for victims of circumstance. It is a challenging road to self–transcendence and development.

No matter who you are, or what your past, you are a worthy person, capable of extraordinary accomplishments. And whether you are parenting alone, or with a partner, it is still your own inner strength and determination that will give you the means to make your life a success and to raise healthy, happy children.

My own two pregnancies and on–going parenting adventures have offered me the opportunity to experience first–hand, the bitter–sweet life of raising children without a partner. Along the road I have faced greater challenges than some and more advantages and opportunities than others. My journey has by no means been easy. But I myself — along with the single mothers I interviewed for this book — have found a direct correlation between the size of the challenge and the amount of personal growth and confidence that resulted. I know that this will be true for you as well.

It has been one of my greatest joys to write SINGLE PREGNANCY

– SINGLE PARENTING. It was born out of a need to overcome the end of a long–term relationship simultaneously with the beginning of my second single pregnancy.

In the beginning, sadness over my loss, together with the fact that I was "hormonally challenged", alone and pregnant seemed more than I could bear. Still, I knew if I was to go through with my pregnancy, I needed to face my fears and rise above them. So, upon making the decision to keep my child, I made a conscious decision to find happiness in my situation and to enjoy each moment of my pregnancy. To help me in that process, I began to write.

Writing quickly became my tool for growth and healing. And as a result, this book was born. Along the way, though I faced so many responsibilities as a single working mother, I found a way to get done what my heart called upon me to do. Hard work and my passion for this project gave me the strength and energy I needed to dedicate hundreds of lunch hours, and many evenings after my children were asleep to complete it. For me, it has been a truly cathartic experience to accomplish this goal. And I am truly grateful for the journey.

I hope that SINGLE PREGNANCY – SINGLE PARENTING will prove to be a meaningful companion on your own journey, contributing insight every step of the way. But most of all, I hope that you too will be inspired to reach for your dreams — and that you find the passion necessary to keep yourself on the path toward realizing each of them.

" Hang on, it's going to be a bumpy ride."
Bette Davis, All About Eve.

Note: When discussing babies and children throughout this book, I have alternated use of the pronouns "he" and "she" as a matter of convenience and as a means to communicate a more personal connection to the "child".

$\mathscr{C}$HAPTER ONE

THE SINGLE PREGNANCY
A REALITY CHECK..

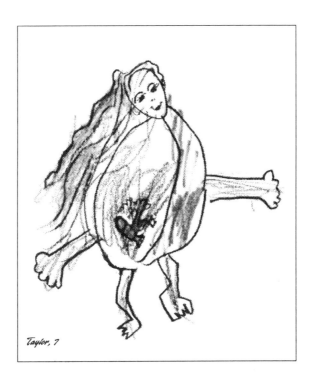

Taylor, 7

OW DID I GET HERE?

If you did not plan to become pregnant, you may be asking yourself how you managed to get yourself into such a predicament. "How did I get here?", "How could I have let this happen?", or "Why me?", may be your own knee jerk reactions to the news of your pregnancy. However, this type of negative "self–talk" is not the kind of reinforcement you need right now.

If you are feeling foolish or disappointed with yourself for getting pregnant, or kicking yourself over your predicament, now is the time to stop! Dwelling upon what you did, what you shouldn't have done, or how foolish you think you were will not change the fact that you are pregnant. Negative self–talk will undermine your pregnancy, your health and possibly even your unborn baby's development. You need a positive attitude now more than you ever have before.

If you find yourself asking "Why me?", turn the question around. Ask yourself "Okay — so now what?"; "What are my options?"; and "How can I turn this into a great experience?" Look to the solutions instead of the problems. This may be hard for you at first, but keep in mind that the messages you give yourself, both positive and negative, will have a lot to do with the your ultimate experience.

To create a positive experience, give yourself positive reinforcement. Even if you don't feel positive right now, *act* your way into correct thinking by giving yourself compliments, rewards, and encouragement. Treat yourself as you would like to have your best friends treat you.

If you already have a positive attitude and are not burdened by negative self–talk, good for you! You have a terrific advantage toward creating a wonderful experience for you and your child, because attitude is fundamental in reaching this goal.

WHAT WE SHARE IN COMMON

My situation is different from yours because (fill in the blank).

What could I possibly share in common with you?

Our "stories" are certainly different. Our social class, ethnic background, education, extended family structure, personalities, religious or spiritual beliefs, and opinions about raising children will differ widely. But we really do have a good deal in common.

Whether you are currently going through a single pregnancy, or are already a single mother, the common denominator between us is that we undoubtedly share many of the same feelings and emotions. No matter what our "stories" are, I'm sure that you will find that we have a lot in common in other ways — not just you and I — but "we" as single mothers in general. It is these similarities that I hope you will look for and relate to.

This book's intention is to create a space for this kind of identification, and to offer useful suggestions for dealing with and enhancing your own unique experience.

While some of the situations will not apply to you, others will strike a familiar cord. Take in, or "borrow" what works or applies, and disregard the rest (or return to it later).

AM I READY FOR THIS?

I wonder if having a baby on my own is realistic. Is this the right thing for me to do?

It's perfectly natural for you to question yourself about your situation. After all, you are taking a major step with this pregnancy. A "healthy hesitation" is to be expected when you are going through such a monumental life change.

Before you go any further you need to figure out if having your baby is the right thing for you to do. Here are some important questions to ask yourself:

- Are you emotionally prepared to meet the challenges of becoming a single–parent.
- Are you mature enough to handle the responsibility?
- Can you afford the medical bills and other expenses of bringing this child into the world?
- Can you support this child monetarily and emotionally?

- Are you willing to make necessary sacrifices for your child?
- Are you stable?
- Do you have any serious problems such as drug or alcohol dependence, emotional instability, or a history of relation ships with abusive men which would adversely affect this child?
- What are your motives in having this child? Are you using a baby to try to solve your unmet needs for love?
- What does having a child mean to you?
- What role, if any, will the father play in his child's life?
- How will you tell your family?

Being honest with yourself is essential. Your answers to practical questions regarding finances, career, emotional stability, etc., will help you get in touch with your feelings and assess your strengths and weaknesses. Your responses may fully support your decision to have your baby on your own. Or, you may find that you are not prepared to have a child at this point in your life. In either case, it will be apparent that there are some problems (big or small) that will need to be addressed during and after your pregnancy.

Once you've identified the problems, you will want to examine your options for solving them.

For example, if you have a demanding career which requires long hours or extended trips, what sacrifices will you be willing or able to make to raise your child? If you are on welfare or government aid, what can you do to become self–supporting? If you are employed but you don't make enough money to take care of a child, what are some things you can do to enhance your earning capacity?

There are many issues you will need to address in terms of their effect on your life and the life of your unborn child, including your relationship with your child's father, your family, and friends. How supportive are they prepared to be and how will this affect your pregnancy and parenting experiences? It is important to look clearly at all the factors involved and not exaggerate your strengths and weak nesses.

Ultimately there is no black or white, right vs. wrong answer to arrive at. Yet this is a momentous decision that will have a lasting impact on many people's lives. Since you will have to live with whatever decision you do make, no matter what other people say or think about your situation, you need to be certain that the choice you make is the right one for you.

Unlike other major decisions — such as buying a house, moving across country, or changing your job — having a baby is irreversible. If you decide down the road that you are not happy with your choice, you can't take the baby back. So it is critical that you really think through your decision and understand what you are getting yourself into.

You will naturally have doubts and concerns about becoming a single mother. Thus, it will surely be easier on you if you resolve these issues at the outset of your pregnancy so that you can feel confident and settled about your choice — regardless of what it is.

FACING THE FEAR

I am frightened by the prospect of being pregnant without a partner to help me through the process. What can I do to make those nine months easier on myself?

Pregnancy is scary enough when you have a partner, so of course it's particularly frightening when you don't. But there are many things you can do to help yourself get through your pregnancy with relative ease.

Once again, look at the messages you're giving yourself. Are you acting in a positive manner, or are you dwelling on negativity and problems? A "pitty–pot mentality" will not serve you well during your pregnancy.

It is not productive for you to dwell on what you don't have (a partner, etc.), your difficulties (not enough money, etc.), your mood (perhaps you are sad or lonely), or other negative feelings. It's what you do about these things that will make the difference.

Give yourself a chance to express your feelings—in your journal or to a friend or therapist. Then focus on the possibilities instead of the impossibilities. Embrace your challenges as opportunities for learning and growth. These actions will go a long way toward making your outlook optimistic and your experience more rewarding.

Other things you can do to feel better about yourself and your pregnancy are to work diligently toward good health (i.e., exercise and diet); take care of your personal appearance; see to your emotional needs (meditation, relaxation, support groups or counceling, etc.); prepare for your baby's arrival (interview doctors, buy the necessities for baby, secure child care if necessary, etc.); and eliminate or reduce the daily stresses in your life. These activities are set forth in more detail throughout this book.

At first it may seem overwhelming to think about all you must do to take care of yourself and your baby's needs without a partner. But if you learn to prioritize, take things one step at a time, look for assistance where possible, and adopt a positive attitude, you will be amazed at what you can accomplish. As you begin to conquer one challenge, and then another, you will gain more confidence in yourself and your abilities.

REACTIONS TO THE NEWS

Carrying a baby in your womb for nine long months without the love and support of a partner can be a challenging experience. Whether you chose to become pregnant, or you have decided to keep your baby after an unplanned pregnancy; you will surely have a wide range of emotions and feelings about your pregnancy. So too will your friends, family, co–workers, employer, and others.

Is it reasonable for me to expect that my family and friends will support my decision to become a single mother?

You will likely find that you receive a variety of different reactions to your solo pregnancy from the people around you — everything from super–positive to super–negative. The reactions you get will largely depend upon each person's values, judgments, religious beliefs, and life experiences — among other things. Keeping that in mind will help you to prepare yourself to accept people's reactions without taking them too personally.

Of course it would be wonderful if your family and friends fully supported you and embraced your decision to be a single–parent. But in *expecting* that reaction, you may just be setting yourself up for disappointment. Be open minded. Accept that some reactions will be supportive and others may not. That's just the way it is when you go against convention and "popular wisdom."

My family/friends do not agree with my decision to keep my baby. They think I am making a mistake. How can I convince them that my decision is the best one for me and my child?

If your friends or family do not approve of your decision, they will probably not change their position just because you would like them to. Your attempt to convince them through lengthy conversations or debates will probably not be successful. So after all points of view have been expressed, it is probably best to drop the subject for a while.

You may feel sad or angry about their reaction or lack of support. After all, you need support now more than ever. Even if you are a strong and confident individual, their negative reaction will likely affect you. But holding on to resentments toward others is harmful to your overall health and well–being. You may need to muster up a lot of courage to let it go and accept that they do not approve of your decision right now.

Give them time to adjust.

People often need time to come to terms with things they do not understand or openly oppose. Hopefully, they will come around when they are ready to accept that you are serious about going through with your pregnancy.

If your family or friends are not willing to accept your decision, you can let your example in parenting your child — and your child itself — show them that having your baby was indeed the right thing for you to do. Most parents (or friends) who initially disapprove cannot resist a beautiful baby once its presence is a reality.

If they remain unwilling to accept your choice — and your child — after she's born, then you will need to create a network of friends who will support you both. A support system may not replace your family or friends, but it will help to fill a void and will provide you with the encouragement you need.

What can I say to someone who is insensitive toward me and my situation?

During my second pregnancy I was asked some blunt and hurtful questions, such as: "Why would you want to do this to yourself?" and "Are you nuts!" While I don't think people meant to be offensive, the tone and sharpness of their questions were unmistakably rude and made me uncomfortable, presenting another obstacle to overcome.

If someone is insensitive toward you, it is likely they won't even be aware that they have come across that way. People can be impulsive and curious by nature and often talk before they think. Even strangers may offer unsolicited comments or questions about your choice to have your baby. Because they are not in your shoes, they may not have empathy toward your situation and may not stop to consider your feelings.

Consider your responses in advance.

One way to protect yourself from other people's negativity is to prepare yourself to deal with it before it comes your way. Try not to expect it, but be aware that it may occur. Take some time to consider your possible responses to criticism or invasive questions.

For example, if someone says "Every child deserves a mom and a dad," imagine yourself responding in a calm and reasonable manner. *"Yes, perhaps they do, but I must deal with my situation as it is and not as I might wish it to be. I will do everything I can to provide my child with positive male role models, and will create a loving and supportive environment."*

Another example of a typical comment might be: "You are going to ruin your future/career." Your response might be: *"My life will not stop because I have this child. In fact, I intend that she will be an addition to my life, not a detraction from it. My professional goals may take longer to reach, but my child does not have to stop me from reaching them. Being a mother is one of my most cherished goals."*

If someone hurts your feelings, especially if they are someone who is close to you, it would be perfectly reasonable for you to let them know how you feel. It's not healthy for you (emotionally or physically) to hold on to hurt or angry feelings To say to them in a calm fashion, *"What you said made me feel uncomfortable and hurt my feelings,"* is okay. In fact, it's a good idea to be honest with people about how you feel.

DON'T WORRY ABOUT WHAT OTHERS THINK

Most of us have a natural desire to please other people. However, some of us are a bit more needy of gaining approval from others than is healthy for us. We worry about what others think of us, and often feel a need to make them happy by doing what they want us to do. We try to live up to their expectations, but inevitably fall short anyway, while making ourselves very unhappy in the process. Forsaking one's own needs to please another can be very painful and unhealthy. We may even lose our own identities along the way.

Although it can be helpful to listen to others — and even apply what you feel is appropriate to your situation — ultimately it is what you think that matters most. Your own instincts are your own best guide. Practice listening to your own inner voice and don't be afraid to make mistakes. Mistakes can be used as turning points to new growth and awareness.

People will undoubtedly judge you harshly as a single woman raising a child or children on your own. Let them have their judgments — you can have your child's love.

A SELFLESS COMMITMENT

Is having a baby out of wedlock selfish or self centered?

When you love your child, strive to provide a safe and nurturing environment, and are willing to make the sacrifices which are necessary to ensure your child's well–being; how can this be selfish? When a mother is deeply committed to her child and is conscientious about her parenting skills, raising a child is one of the most selfless things she can do.

UNSOLICITED ADVICE

People are always giving me advice about my pregnancy, or about parenting. How do I know who to listen to?

People just love to give free advice — even when you don't ask for it. "If I were you...", "This is what you need to do...", etc. Ultimately, what works well for one person, may be a disaster for someone else. A good rule of thumb is to be open–minded and willing to try out new ideas. Keep what works, and throw out the rest.

Be sure to pay attention to the source of the advice. If it's someone whose values and judgment you respect, you'll listen more attentively than you would to somebody whose own life is a mess. Not even the experts agree on what is best, so learn to rely on your own intuition — bolstered by input from your experience, your doctor, your reading, and other mothers.

"IF ONLY I HAD A HUSBAND"

If you have said to yourself "If only I had a husband", consider yourself to be in good company. This is a normal reaction when contemplating having a baby without a partner. I have uttered these words many times, believing that life would be easier for my sons and me if I had a partner to share the load. This may well be the truth, but it has not been my lot in life to know. The reality is that it is not yours either — at least for now. Still, it's normal to get caught up in the fantasy of imagining what we think we want. However, it will not serve you or your child to dwell too long or too hard upon what you do not have, or to compare your reality against some ideal image.

To make your parenting experience the best one possible; it is important to focus on what you do have and to see the good and wonderful in your own situation as it is. Even a person of little means — and perhaps big problems — who has love, health and warmth in their heart has much for which to be grateful.

Gratitude will transform your perspective. It can help you to accept what you must, change what you can, and be patient with the often painstaking process of transformation.

Don't give up on a future love.

Don't give up on a future love, a father for your child, or a better career if that's what you want. On the contrary, take care of and nurture yourself so that you're in top shape physically, emotionally, mentally, and spiritually. Then when the time is right and opportunities present themselves, you'll be prepared to make the most of them.

We all want and need love, but must first receive it from ourselves. If you don't already possess a strong sense of self — get one!

Learn to like yourself, to appreciate who you are and the many blessings in your life. Utilize the ideas in this book to help you in this area if you are feeling "stuck" wanting what you don't have and not enjoying what you do have. Take care of business today — live in the moment — and tomorrow will take care of itself.

MAKING DO WITHOUT A PARTNER

As a single–parent, you will become the back–bone of your family. Without Dad's assistance your child's entire life will rest in your hands alone. And even if Dad chooses to provide love, emotional and/or financial support; the daily responsibilities of caring for your child will belong to you.

It's so easy to get caught up in the fantasy of what you think your baby will be like. You may be thinking about how cute, cuddly, warm and wonderful he will be — and how much love you will share together. But have you considered some of the more challenging realities?

Without a partner, you will be the one walking the floor all hours of the night with a colicky baby — or holding your child in the wake of a nightmare. When your child is sick, you will be the one to take time off from work to get him to the doctor and to comfort him through a difficult night. And as he grows, new challenges will unfold. You will be the "heavy" when he doesn't want to eat his vegetables or do his homework. And some of you will have to decide between paying a bill and buying your child some new shoes.

There will be a myriad of conflicts between your child's needs and your own. And as he grows, the responsibilities will only increase: picking the baby up from day care by 6:00pm when you don't get off from work before 6:00pm; attending teacher–parent conferences when you need to be at work; finding time to attend a school play; getting your child to baseball practice or gymnastics, etc. These are just a few examples. Are you prepared for these challenges?

Such challenges are the typical, day-to-day things every mother must deal with — even the married ones. Will you have help in these situations? Will family and friends be there to support you, or will you be completely on your own? Will your child's father be willing or able to assist you with the day-to-day aspects of raising your child? These are all very important things to consider as you contemplate the birth of your child.

ASKING FOR HELP

It's sometimes difficult to ask for help.

During and after your pregnancy, you will likely find that self–sufficiency becomes the norm. In fact, you'll be amazed by all that you're able to handle. But asking for help from family and friends is also essential. While it's easy to say "Don't do it alone, ask for help," it can be difficult to reach out to others — particularly if they're initially opposed your decision — and especially if you're very independent.

In the early days of my parenting adventure, I depended way too much upon myself for anything and everything I needed. It didn't matter what I was going through at any given time. I felt that if I asked for help it was a sign of weakness.

In retrospect, it seems odd to me now that though there were loving arms reaching out to help, I couldn't accept that help. When people openly offered to assist me, I would say "Oh no, that's okay, I can do it myself." Stubbornness and pride, as well as the fear of appearing incompetent, stood in my way. How much more difficult I made things on myself over those first few years! I held this crazy belief that if I asked for help *they* would say "I told you so... you can't do this on your own!" My inability to reach out was hurting me and my son and I didn't even know it.

Finally, a friend pointed out that "Some of the most selfish people in this world are those who won't let anybody in to help them." This struck me as very logical and perhaps even true.

Had I actually been selfish by not allowing friends and family to give me the gift of love? After all, helping another is ultimately an act of love and concern. And in my life, there were so many people who really loved me. I saw that I was needlessly putting more stress upon myself by maintaining the attitude that "I can do this myself!" And I was also becoming more and more bitter about my burdens.

Learning to reach out.

It is only natural that we come to rely more and more upon

ourselves to take care of business. This can be wonderful and empowering. There is a great deal of satisfaction in being (or becoming) self–sufficient. But, a middle ground is necessary. A balance between self–sufficiency and openness to allowing others to help us is essential.

When I was a new mother, it was really scary to reach out for help and to accept it with grace. In fact, it is sometimes still difficult for me. But I stretch my boundaries anyway. I was determined to change my belief about what asking for help meant to me. I began in small measures to allow others to be there for me and found that they were happy and willing to help out once I let them. By the way — nobody ever said "I told you so" or considered me to be weak.

As you go about your life, solving problems, handling your pregnancy, raising your kids, and blazing the trail so–to–speak, you may find that asking others to help you enhances your relationships and bonds you and your child more closely with those around you. Allow the loving arms of others to be there for you.

Even though I have a very supportive family, I still find there's a void they can't fill.

While you allow others to help you throughout your pregnancy and after the birth of your child, it is natural that you may still have an empty feeling. There may be a relationship void which they cannot fill.

The absence of a partner may cause you to feel sad and lonely, particularly during pregnancy. And after your baby is born, the lack of support from a partner may be frustrating and deeply disappointing.

Having a loving partner to share in the experience of pregnancy and parenting can be very comforting in a way that friends and family cannot be. Assuming they do not overwhelm you, such feelings of loss or lack are normal.

If you experience such feelings and emotions, you should not be expected to ignore them. Simply accepting their presence will help you through the process. As stated earlier, acknowledge that you feel sad and then express your emotions. Write about them. Share your feelings with a friend or loved one. Go ahead and get it out. I like to say to my friends (and myself) "You can go there — just don't stay there too long." If you find that you cannot shake these feelings on your own, it might be a good time to look into counseling.

Filling the void.

Though you may have that "empty" feeling, you can still find happiness and fulfillment — even without a partner to share the blessings and burdens. It may not always be easy, but it will be helpful if you focus on the things you *can* do to enhance your experience, instead of sitting around feeling sorry for yourself. Try some of the processes and activities suggested throughout this book to get back on track.

I found, during difficult times, that it was very helpful to create and maintain platonic male friendships in addition to my female friendships. Jennifer, the single mother of two agrees. "Having male energy around has been an important asset to my life and to my children. I feel comforted just knowing I can call up and get the 'male point of view.' These friendships have also helped me to feel less lonely when I missed my ex–husband."

Dependency is not the answer either.

It is important to allow other people to help you when you need it. But there is the other extreme which needs to be looked at as well. If you are too dependent on other people to help you, and to take care of you (and your child), this may be an indication that some adjustments need to be made in your life. It is great to ask for, and receive help (in whatever form). At the same time, you need to be responsible for your own life. Assuming you are healthy, you can't make other people responsible to carry your weight.

It can be tempting to fall into a trap of allowing other people to take care of you. It appears to simplify life and make things less painful. However, you lose some of your own identity and pride as the price for greater ease.

If you find that this scenario describes you, you might ask yourself what you can do to take more responsibility for your life. For example, if your parents are supporting you, what can you do to improve your financial picture? Are you going to school to learn a new skill? If you are constantly complaining to a friend, consider what you can do to take more responsibility for changing your circumstances.

It is wise to create a balance between receiving assistance and taking responsibility, not only for ourselves, but for our children. Our children need to see us taking responsibility for our lives so that they will learn to assume responsibility for their own lives.

WORDS OF WISDOM

While not much exists in the marketplace in the way of pregnancy books written specifically for the single woman, there are a few. I've also listed a few good books which address single–parenting:

- *Single Mothers by Choice: A Guidebook For Single Women Who Are Considering or Have Chosen Motherhood,* by Jane Mattes (Random House/Times Books)
- *Two Of Us Make A World: The Single Mother's Guide to Pregnancy, Childbirth, and the First Year,* by Prudence and Sherill Tippins (An Owl Book/Henry Holt and Company)
- *Joy of Single Mothering: Reassuring Answers to Your Most Challenging Concerns,* by Andrea Engber (Bob Adams)
- *Solo Parenting – Your Essential Guide: How to Find the Balance Between Parenthood and Personhood,* by Kathleen McCoy (A Plume Book/New American Library)
- The Hite Report on the Family: Growing up Under Patriarchy, by researcher, Shere Hite (Grove Press)

Some books for children living in single–parent families are:

- *Tell Me No Lies,* by Hila Colman (Crown Publishers)
- *It's Not the End of the World,* by Judy Blume (Bradbury Press)
- *My Kind of Family: A Book for Kids in Single– Parent Homes* (Waterfront Books)
- *The Boys' and Girls' Book About One Parent Families* (Bantam Books)
- *Do I Have A Daddy? (Yo tengo papa?)* (Morning Glory Press)
- *How It Feels When Parents Divorce* (Knopf)
- *How It Feels to Be Adopted* (Knopf)

- *How It Feels When a Parent Dies* (Knopf)
- *Heather Has Two Mommies* (Ayson Publications)

✐ Pioneer Woman

I dreamt I was a pioneer lady
grand and tall – stronger than ten armies
disheveled and dusty
blazing trails
climbing hills, moving mountains
every now and again
fixing broken wheels
 of my wagon
all by myself –
The uncharted course of my destination
rugged and rough as it was
often sent me wild Indians
who frightened me until I learned
not to fear what I didn't understand
but to look upon the Indians as friends
and symbols of opportunity
to be stronger for the wear
and to find my way
along the trail
and then I looked at the baby in my arms
and realized
I wasn't dreaming at all

I CAN DO THIS!

Despite set–backs and difficulties, over the years I have happily discovered that my ability to raise my children on my own and without a partner far exceeded my own initial expectations of myself; and indeed even surpassed those of others who know me (some of whom thought I was doomed to failure). For my part, I never considered that I couldn't do it. But I didn't know I could do it so well.

You will take spills until you learn to walk.

Much like a baby who is learning to walk, I tripped a few times and fell down; but I kept getting back up, determined to make it work. Can you imagine what would happen if all babies gave up just because they couldn't walk the first few times they tried? They don't have the slightest notion that they can't do it. They just keep trying until they master their little feet.

Like a baby learning to walk, you will need to keep getting back up until you learn to walk — both during your pregnancy and after. Metaphorically speaking, once you master walking, you will then have the challenge of learning to run, skip, jump, ride a bike, etc.

You may still question yourself and worry about your abilities. You may experience feelings of guilt or loneliness. You may be scraping by on limited finances, or have any number of other worries. These are the spills you will take as you learn to walk. Every mother (even if she's married) has them. Keep pushing yourself to get up and overcome your problems. With practice, you will be amazed at what you can do when you are determined. The possibilities are endless.

In my discussions with many of the women I interviewed for this book, I noticed an interesting phenomena. Though they were accomplishing great feats of their own; they managed to take them in stride and believed that other women had far greater challenges. While none of these women had anticipated having to deal with so many problems, they naturally rose to the occasion when the challenges were presented. The harder the challenge the higher we climb. For most of us, it is our natural instinct.

You will find that you can do things you never imagined you could do. Even the so–called "impossible" becomes possible when you have no choice but to get the job done. As you discover hidden capabilities, "I can't do it" will fade from your vocabulary.

When there's not another person there to do it for you (whatever "it" may be,) you will learn to rise to the occasion. Without a doubt, you will find that there will be times (probably many times,) when you do not have any choice but to figure out a creative way to solve a difficult problem.

CHAPTER TWO

SINGLE PREGNANCY – SINGLE PARENTING – AND SOCIETY

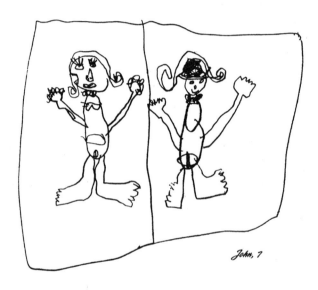

John, 7

CONTROVERSIAL ISSUE

There is no doubt that we have come a long way since the days when a young, unmarried woman "with child" would be ostracized by her community. Then she was either sent away from home and forced to give up her baby for adoption; or made to suffer a life threatening, back–street abortion. While such blatant rejection of a single pregnant woman is not so prevalent today, there still remains a stigma attached to an unmarried woman having a child.

THE DAN QUAYLE PERSPECTIVE

As you may recall, several years ago former Vice President, Dan Quayle made a widely publicized statement about "Murphy Brown", a fictional character in a hit television series, who became pregnant and chose to become a single mother. "It doesn't help matters," Quayle complained, when "a character who supposedly epitomizes today's intelligent, highly paid professional woman" is portrayed as "mocking the importance of fathers by bearing children alone, and calling it just another lifestyle choice."

Mr. Quayle went on to blame the 1992 Los Angeles riots on the "poverty of values" that Murphy Brown's out–of–wedlock parenting represented. Mr. Quayle's comments triggered anger, jokes and a heated national debate over "family values". Single mothers were caught smack in the middle of the debate.

Does pregnancy outside of marriage "mock" the importance of fathers as some might suggest?

Many believe that a woman's choice to have a child outside of marriage is not meant to be a statement on the importance of fathers. Rather, it is a choice made at a given time, under given circumstances, which precluded the father's role as an active parent. Actually, most single mothers agree that a father is very important to a child. But for any number of reasons, sometimes "he" is not the deciding factor when making the choice to have a child. Does that mean we "mock" fathers? Not at all.

THE DEBATE CONTINUES

On one side of the debate are those who support a woman's right to choose to have children outside of marriage. On the other side, are many religious leaders, politicians, social critics, and other groups who agree with the Quayle perspective. It is interesting to note, however, that many of these people, while they oppose single–parenting, also oppose abortions. Nothing short of conventional marriage satisfies some people where having babies is concerned. Such people believe that an out–of–wedlock pregnancy is inappropriate under any circumstances.

Many of those who side with the Quayle perspective consider unmarried pregnant women to be sexually promiscuous, selfish, and immoral. Others assume that unwed pregnant women, particularly younger women, become pregnant in order to collect government aid. There are also those who assume all single mothers are losers, drug addicts/alcoholics, teenage misfits and the like.

WHOSE FAMILY VALUES?

Indeed, many critics will argue that a single–parent family is a deficient family structure. They point to a decline in family values – – as if *they* are the arbiters of family values and morality. It doesn't matter that you may have chosen to become pregnant, or that you are a solid person with decent values. Single mothers are generally assumed to be morally deficient; and the decision to have a baby out–of–wedlock is considered wrong under any circumstances.

The media, including television, film, books, and magazines often perpetuate this negative image. Even President Clinton, himself the son of a single mother, is quoted as saying "The epidemic of illegitimacy is our most serious social problem..."

Is illegitimacy our most serious social problem as Clinton suggests?

It seems unreasonable and over–reaching to say that "illegitimacy", is, in and of itself, our most serious social problem. Rather, they are issues such as lack of education; poverty; substance abuse; lack of positive male role models, on all levels of society from fathers to Presidents; poor parenting skills; and often the sheer laziness a parent displays toward a child which contributes most to our most serious social problems.

While we cannot deny that these problems exist in some single–parent families, it is clear that they also exist in two–parent families. Furthermore, while some single mothers may be unfit role models who do not teach family values to their children, one cannot assume that *all* single mothers lack decent family values — anymore than one can assume that *all* married parents possess these qualities. Family values are possessed by people — not by institutions such as marriage. Under any family structure, single or otherwise, the underlying problems, as discussed, need to be addressed to effectuate change.

In the meantime, there are many single mothers who are doing a fine job of raising their children. According to researcher and author, Shere Hite, "The great majority of single mothers, whom fundamentalist groups try to put on the defensive, can indeed be proud of the excellent job they are doing in bringing up their children, often despite financial hardship."

Contrary to what we hear in the media, there exist many exemplary single mothers who anonymously go about their lives, raising healthy, well–adjusted children. They exist in little towns and big cities. But likely, we don't hear very much about these single–parent success stories because they don't make for sensational news and because their presence contradicts a wide–spread belief that is as old as patriarchy itself.

So what can be done about the problems and the perceptions?

The issues of troubled families need to be addressed on a larger, perhaps even global scale. As a culture we need to find a way to solve the underlying problems of poverty, addiction and illiteracy, etc., so that these problems are not passed from one generation to the next.

While I don't claim to have better answers than our political and religious leaders espouse, I do believe that more effective answers would be gained by effective dialogue and movement toward "problem solving" rather than constantly complaining about the "problem".

Single–parenting is here to stay.

Single–parenting is happening whether we like it or not, and it's not going to go away. Until we start to address "now what" and find solutions for the greater problems of illiteracy, poverty, drug abuse, alcoholism, child abuse, "dead–beat dads", etc., we won't make any progress toward change.

Though I don't necessarily believe government should be responsible to subsidize all programs for all people, I firmly believe that if we don't spend money on intervention programs now, society will pay a greater price later on. Although some helpful programs currently exist, many women are not adequately informed of the existence of them by social workers and other government agencies. Furthermore, Congress is threatening to cut a large number of the federal programs that do exist. They include programs that offer child care, job training, money, abortions, and food to women below the poverty line.

AN OUNCE OF PREVENTION...

Notwithstanding the view held by some that these programs *need* to be cut, I believe many programs *need* to be more vigorously promoted and encouraged to ensure better opportunities for mothers and children. These include accessible, mandatory early education for pregnant women who are on government aid, including parenting, prenatal, and postpartum classes. These classes should also be made more readily available to low–to–middle income women, on a sliding scale, according to ability to pay.

Additionally, we must create more viable options to help women get off government aid, including vocational and job–related preparation programs. Women need to be encouraged to take personal responsibility for their lives, but we need to support them through programs which offer hope for a viable future. We also need better tax breaks for single–parent families; more access to affordable or subsidized substance abuse programs; and access to counseling programs that focus on family dynamics. And we need stricter child support enforcement laws. Although many child support enforcement agencies are finally beginning to crack down on "dead–beat dads", the system continues to be inadequate to meet the needs of children and the mothers who *need* to feed them *today*.

Advocacy – letting your voice be heard.

While you may not be able to change the big picture all by yourself, you can get involved in creating change through advocacy. Write to politicians, governmental agencies, the media, etc. If you have something to say, say it! Let your voice be heard. If you do nothing, but find things to complain about, you are not contributing to the solution.

On a personal level, in your everyday life, there are many effective ways for you to improve your chances of raising a healthy, happy, secure child. We will talk about many of them in the coming chapters.

AN ANTIQUATED IDEA – "ILLEGITIMACY"

Possibly more disturbing than any debate over the issues of single pregnancies and single–parenting is the fact our society still considers a child to be "illegitimate" if there is not a marriage to the father to "legitimatize" the child. This practice sends the message that we need a man and a marriage to make our children equal to others. Nonsense! By their very nature, our babies are "legitimate" *even* when we bring them into this world without a marriage certificate.

The term "illegitimate" has been a legal standard for centuries with ramifications on inheritance issues. But the use of this term today is as inappropriate as calling African American's "Negroes". The term is antiquated and has negative connotations. Perhaps in time we will phase out this word within our legal system in favor of a term which does not insult us and our children.

The term "bastard" is also inappropriate. Referring to a father-

less child as a bastard is as cruel and unacceptable as describing someone by a racial epithet. What message does a child receive when he
or she hears this? How does this make them feel about themselves?
By continuing to label children born out–of–wedlock in this degrad-
ing and hurtful manner, society continues to fuel the flame of prejudice and intolerance, further undermining the single–parent family.

When making the decision to have a baby on your own, you
might want to think about these value judgments. How will they affect you and your child? Are you prepared to face and overcome
such attitudes and labels if they come your way?

STATISTICAL FACTS

Over the last three decades, the number of unmarried women
venturing through single pregnancies has risen dramatically both in
the United States and abroad. According to the U.S. Census Bureau's
1994 statistics (the most recent available bureau study) 26 percent of
total births in the United States were to single mothers. In simple
numbers, this means that one in four children are born to unmarried
women. Thus, with over one million single women giving birth to
babies each year in our country alone, the importance of issues related to "single pregnancies" are evident. Also evident in our society
are the issues related to single–parent households (as distinguished
from single pregnancies).

Today over seventeen million households are headed by single–
parents (mothers and fathers.) Of those, approximately 90 percent
are headed by single women. There is little indication that this trend
will change in the near future. To the contrary, with each passing
year, the overall number of single–parent households continues to
rise. In fact, over the last thirty years the number of single–parent
households has more than tripled in this country.

SOME NOT–SO–GOOD NEWS

**What do studies indicate about children who are raised in
single parent households?**

According to David Elwood, the Assistant Secretary of Planning and Evaluation for the Department of Health and Human Services, nearly 73 percent of children from single–parent families will be in poverty at some point during their childhood. While only 20 percent of children in two–parent families will experience poverty.

It is appalling that any child would ever be subjected to poverty, but the sad reality is that many are — particularly those in single–parent households. This problem has a good deal to do with the fact that a woman's earning capacity continues to be significantly less than a man's. And when she lacks a higher education, her ability to earn even a decent living is further impaired. The problems faced by many children who grow up in poverty are compounded by the fact that far too many men refuse to meet the moral and legal obligation they have to support the children whom they father. These factors, among others, undoubtedly contribute significantly to the problems these children face.

In a study conducted at Cornell University, it was determined that children growing up in single–parent households are more likely to experience a variety of behavioral problems. Those problems include hyperactivity, withdrawal, school misbehavior, absenteeism, dropping out, involvement in socially alienated peer groups, smoking, drinking, early sexual activities, drugs, violence, vandalism, and criminal acts, among others. Another study indicated that children who are raised in single–parent families experience higher than average levels of youth suicide, low intellectual and educational performance, and higher than average rates of mental illness.

"Not me — not my kid!"

These studies, and others like them, are so alarming as to be frightening. How scary it is to think that our children could face such difficulties! We want to deny it. We want to believe it couldn't happen to us — "Not me – Not my kid!" "I am (or will be) a 'better' parent than 'those' parents who produce maladjusted or impoverished children. I am 'different'."

Our natural inclination may be to bury our head in the sand when we hear these terrible statistics and potential problems. We do not want to face the fear, the guilt, or the possibility that we cannot provide for our children or protect them from social ills and temptations. But being aware is important. Understanding that certain problems occur more frequently in single–parent households can motivate you to be a more conscientious parent. Or it can discourage you from undertaking the challenge if you are not yet prepared to meet it well.

THE FLIP SIDE
OR...THE GOOD NEWS

Though children typically do better in a (healthy) two–parent environment — in contrast to the negative stereotypes we hear so much about — as a single–parent you can do a terrific job of raising a child who thrives.

The fact that you are a single–parent will certainly have an affect on your child, but it doesn't necessarily have to be a negative one. Even some experts will tell you that many problems found in children of single–parents are more the result of poor parenting skills or limited resources, rather than the lack of a second parent.

In "The Hite Report on the Family," Shere Hite, challenges the nostalgia of the two–parent nuclear family and an idealized past by analyzing the nature of all kinds of families — both traditional and nontraditional. Hite's data indicates that there are beneficial effects for the majority of children living in single–parent families, including:

- Men raised by single mothers tend to have better relationships with women later in life.
- With the rise in single working mothers, children's respect for their mothers has increased significantly.
- Children are sometimes better off in an environment of equaity — therefore, a single–parent family is often preferable to a two–parent family where inequality between the parents exists.

Furthermore, Hite's finding include the premise that the current family crisis is really a sign of transformation and not collapse. She indicates that the current slogan "preservation of family values" really means not preservation of love in the family, but preservation of the hierarchical family with the father at its head. Furthermore, Hite believes that as society advances and changes, women are democratizing and bringing equity to an institution that was never democratized before. Naturally this makes many people uncomfortable.

In order to raise your child successfully, you need to look at your parenting skills and other factors which will influence your child's development. Your ability to love, nurture, support, and encourage high self–esteem within your child are critical factors for success. Keeping your eye on these and other emotional/behavioral indicators will help you navigate to your desired destination: enjoying the process of raising a healthy, happy, emotionally secure child.

What is the impact to my child in having only one parent?

While statistically we've already seen that in our single–parent family there are some odds against our children, these are not necessarily hard and fast rules. Despite such statistics, and as a result of our diligent efforts and good parenting skills, we can indeed raise a positive, well–adjusted child. But the question may still remain: "What is the impact to my child in having only one parent?" This is not a questions which can easily be answered, if at all.

Because each situation is unique, there is no way to predict just how your child will be affected by growing up without a father. Every child will be raised with a different set of circumstances, including their support system, available economic resources, and the influences of their community, school, friends, family, etc. Additionally, the quality of your parenting skills will differ from others', and the individual personality of your child will influence their experience as well.

While the absence of a loving father will certainly affect your child, the success you achieve in raising her is more a result of the quality of your parenting skills than the quantity of parents living in your home.

Dr. Leah Klungness, a New York psychologist and single mother of two, says: "When you have difficulties with your children, don't automatically assume or let others tell you that it is because your children are being raised in a broken home. Don't listen to those who make dire predictions about fatherless boys. They are wrong."

Whether there are two parents in the home or only one is not the determining factor for a child's mental health. Good child–rearing depends more upon the commitment and abilities of the person or persons doing the job. If you have good parenting skills, and give your child a strong foundation of love, emotional support, encouragement, and the other essential ingredients that go into creating a healthy, happy, productive individual, then she will be more likely to flourish into a loving and nurturing adult.

It is perhaps true that a single–parent must go the extra distance and work harder to do the best job possible — and make no mistake about it, parenting is a full–time job. But there are millions of women today who are proving their ability to raise a child on their own and doing a very good job of it.

WELL–KNOWN SINGLE MOTHERS AND CHILDREN OF SINGLE MOTHERS

Some of the following single mothers had children outside of marriage. Some divorced, were widowed, or adopted a child. Whether briefly or for a good portion of their lives, each of these courageous women were destined to meet the challenges and difficulties of single–parenting:

- Golda Meir, former Prime Minister, Israel
- Jane Wallace, TV journalist
- Marianne Williamson, writer, lecturer
- Carol Moseley–Braun, Senator
- Cleopatra, Egyptian Queen/head of army
- Theodora, Byzantine Empress
- Jacqueline Kennedy Onassis, former first lady, editor
- Virginia Kelly, mother of Jacqueline Kennedy Onassis
- Linda Rondstadt, singer
- Gypsy Rose Lee, entertainer
- Chrissie Hynde, singer/musician (The Pretenders)
- Margaret Meade, anthropologist
- Maya Angelou, civil rights activist, author, actress, film director and producer
- Catherine Deneuve, actress
- Ingrid Bergman, actress
- Isadora Duncan, innovative dancer in the early 1900's
- Mary Wollstonecraft, feminist, writer
- Tasha Tudor, illustrator/children's book author

- Whoopi Goldberg, comedian, actress
- Dorothy Thompson, journalist
- Augusta Christine Savage, sculptor
- Margaret Sanger, pioneer in contraception education - in 1913- brought contraception to America
- George Sand (born Amantine–Lucile–Aurore Dupin), most widely read novelist in the mid to late 1800's
- Harriet Strong, inventor of water conservation techniques
- Vivienne Westwood, fashion designer
- Ann London Scott, activist
- Georgia Lee Mitt Lusk, Congresswoman
- Hedda Hopper, columnist
- Frieda Segelke Miller, labor reformer
- Mabel Walker Willebrandt, hailed as "First Lady in Law"
- Frances Marion, screenwriter
- Rosie O'Donnell
- Madonna

Some famous, and even heroic people have been raised by single mothers. They include:

- Bill Clinton, President
- Newt Gingrich, politician
- Alexander Haig, Jr., Former White House Chief of Staff and Secretary of State
- Oprah Winfrey, talk show host, producer, actress
- Tom Cruise, actor
- Ed Bradley, news correspondent and co–editor of 60 Minutes
- Caroline Kennedy, daughter of John F. Kennedy
- John F. Kennedy, Jr., son of John F. Kennedy
- Jack Nicholson, actor
- John Lennon, musician, writer, singer
- Lucille Ball, actress, producer
- James Earl Jones, actor
- Patty Duke, actress
- Audrey Hepburn, actress
- Mickey Rooney, actor
- George Washington, 1st President
- Sir Isaac Newton, mathematician & natural philosopher
- Jodie Foster, actress, director
- Ricky Henderson, baseball player–Texas Rangers
- Alan Greenspan, economist
- Lauren Hutton, actress, talk show host
- Louis Armstrong, jazz musician
- Carol Burnett, actress, comedian
- Les Brown, public speaker and author
- Mary Higgins Clark, author

CHAPTER THREE

STAGES OF PREGNANCY

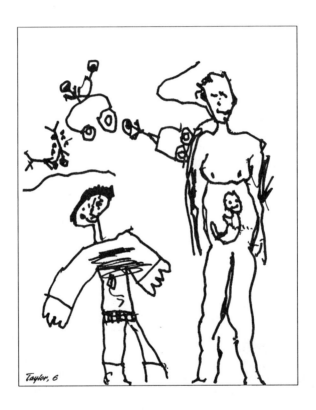

Taylor, 6

onception occurs approximately two weeks after the first day of your last menstrual period. The egg and sperm fuse together to produce one cell. In the first weeks after conception, this single cell rapidly divides forming a hollow ball of cells that attaches itself to the womb. Some of the cells will become the embryo; the rest will become the placenta.

In the first trimester (3 months,) the embryo takes shape and all the organs are formed. In the last 6 months, the fetus grows and matures.

DEVELOPMENT STAGES OF THE FETUS

1–3 weeks: Or about one week after the first period is missed, the embryo is 1/10 of an inch long and has an oval shape.

3 weeks: Nervous system begins to develop and the spinal cord is forming. The embryo is becoming more oval in shape, and a head and tail become more discernable. A tubular heart begins to form and beat – but it is too faint to hear at this time.

4 weeks: Lungs, liver, stomach and intestines begin to form.

5 weeks: Your future child is still an embryo. It is about 1/4 inch long, already has a two–lobed brain. Arms and leg buds appear.

6 weeks: Diaphragm forms — separating chest and stomach.

7 weeks: Measurable brain waves begin. The embryo is called a fetus at the seventh – eighth week.

8 weeks: Facial features are formed. By the end of eight weeks, the fingers, toes, ears, and eyes have begun to form. The fetus is about 7/8ths to one inch long and weighs approximately 1/30 of an ounce. The head is disproportionately large because of the size of the developing brain — and the abdomen seems large because of the growing liver. The pituitary, adrenal and thyroid glands are present.

9 weeks: The organs are established, and will undergo only fine differentiation from this point forward.

10 weeks: Brain and muscles can now communicate.

11 weeks: Vocal cords form.

End of the third month: By the end of the third month, the fetus is two to three inches long and weighs less than an ounce. Nails form on the fingers and toes. The male or female sex organs begin to develop, and the bones begin to calcify. The skeletal muscles begin to work as well — and the fetus can move in response to local pressure. The tooth buds are formed in the mouth. Breathing movements begin and the fetus starts to swallow amniotic fluid. The muscles of the intestines contract and relax — as if digesting food.

The second trimester: The second trimester is devoted primarily to maturation of the organs. By the fourth month, the fetus is 4–5 inches long and weighs about 3 ounces. About this time, the fetus moves spontaneously — but is generally too small for most mothers to feel — although some fetuses may be large enough to be felt.

By the fifth month, the fetus is about 6 inches long and weighs about one–half pound. The baby is now strong enough to make its presence felt. The baby's movement is known as "quickening." At this stage, the baby's body is covered with fine hair called "lanugo" and coarse hair appears on the head.

The third trimester: By the beginning of the third the baby is fully developed. And the last three months are devoted to the baby's growth. The fetus is about 10 inches long and weighs 1–2 pounds by the seventh month. The skin is thin, red, and wrinkled — and becomes covered with "vernix," a protective, fatty, white, sticky substance composed of skin cells, lanugo, and oily skin secretions.

If the baby were born at this time (around the seventh month,) with proper medical care, the baby would have a 50/50 chance of survival — though some statistics cite a higher rate of survival. Babies born at this early stage can respond to sound, taste, and light.

If the baby is born during the eighth month, her chance of survival increases to 90%. By this time, she is about 10–12 inches long and weighs 3–4 pounds.

The final month: During the ninth month, a substance called "surfactant" develops and lines the lungs, allowing them to expand easily. Fat is stored, and its deposition under the skin smooths out the wrinkles. Much of the lanugo disappears. At this time, the baby is approximately 14–16 inches long and weighs 7–8 pounds.

Note: Throughout your pregnancy, keep in mind how important your nutritional needs are to both you and your growing fetus. *See* Chapter Four, *Eating Healthy*, page 56.

PHYSICAL/EMOTIONAL CHANGES DURING PREGNANCY

You may (or may not) experience any number of the conditions described on the following pages at some point during the course of your pregnancy. But every pregnancy is different, and every woman will have different experiences.

The first trimester (the first through third months)

- Menstruation stops. Though it is normal for some women to have a slight stain when her period would have been due, or when the fertilized egg implants in the uterus.
- Changes in your breasts. Fullness, swelling, heaviness, tenderness, and/or tingling; darkening of the pigmented area surrounding the nipple (the areola). The sebaceous (sweat) glands in the areola become enlarged (like goose bumps). Veins may begin to appear under the skin (on the breasts, abdomen and legs) as blood supply to the breasts increases (this occurs more prominently in fair–skinned women).
- Frequent need to urinate.
- Nausea, vomiting, and/or excessive salivation.
- Light–headedness or dizziness.
- Fatigue and sleepiness (slight or extreme).
- Mood swings, depression, bouts of crying.
- Indigestion, heartburn, bloating, flatulence, constipation.
- Food cravings, and sometimes aversions to certain foods.
- Increase/decrease in sexual appetite.
- Occasional headaches.
- Aggravated allergies — though some women experience relief from them during pregnancy.
- Complexion problems, dry – itchy skin (drink lots of water to hydrate the skin) — though some women have a "radiant" complexion during pregnancy.
- Dry, coarse, lackluster or limp hair. Though for some, their hair never looked better.
- Usually around the third month: increased appetite.
- Toward the end of your first trimester, your clothes may begin

to get a little tight around the waist, stomach and breasts.
• Toward the end of your first trimester: stretch marks may begin to appear on the breasts, abdomen, hips and/or thighs. About 90% of women get these dreaded marks — though they will gradually fade after delivery.

The second trimester (the fourth through sixth months)

• Around the fourth month: a decrease, or end, to nausea and vomiting — though some women do not get relief. In a very few women, nausea — with or without vomiting — may begin.
• Continuing increase in appetite.
• Continuing fatigue for some — though many women may have more energy after adjusting to pregnancy.
• Decrease in need to urinate as frequently.
• Breasts continue to enlarge — though the tenderness usually decreases.
• Indigestion, heartburn, flatulence, and/or constipation may continue.
• Hemorrhoids.
• Occasional headaches.
• Light–headedness or dizziness.
• As your second trimester progresses, you may experience forgetfulness — it's common to have trouble concentrating, or forget even the most simple things — even for well–organized, intelligent women.
• Gum bleeds.
• Possible nosebleeds, nasal congestion, ear stuffiness.
• Swelling of feet and ankles, and possibly hands and face.
• Varicose veins in legs. Leg cramps toward the fifth–six month.
• In some women, (approximately 1%–2%) elevated blood pressure occurs.
• Increased pulse (heart rate) – toward the fifth–sixth month.
• Backache.
• Toward the fifth–sixth month, sleeping position may become a bit more uncomfortable.
• Skin pigmentation changes on the face and/or abdomen.
• For a few women, particularly slimmer women, fetal move-

ment may be felt around the fourth month, but for most it occurs around the fifth month.

- Expanding waist–line.
- Increase/decrease in sexual appetite.
- Increasing whitish vaginal discharge (leukorrhea).
- Lower abdominal achiness (caused by stretching ligaments supporting the uterus). This usually occurs more toward your fifth–sixth month.

The third trimester (The seventh through ninth months)

- Stronger and more frequent fetal activity — becoming more regular around the eight month. Around the ninth month, there will be less kicking and more squirming as the baby has less room to move around.
- Increase or loss of appetite.
- Increasing fatigue — though some women have bursts of energy, or alternating periods of each toward the latter month or so.
- Indigestion, heartburn, flatulence, constipation (increasing around the eight month).
- Hemorrhoids.
- Occasional headaches.
- Light–headedness or dizziness.
- Shortness of breath — increasing around the eighth–ninth months as the uterus crowds the lungs — but which should ease up when the baby drops.
- Forgetfulness.
- Clumsiness (increasing the risk of falling). Toward the ninth month, more difficulty getting around, awkward gait.
- Gum bleeds.
- Possible nosebleeds, nasal congestion, ear stuffiness.
- Swelling of feet and ankles, and possibly hands and face. This will increase in the final month.
- Increasingly heavy leukorrhea — a whitish vaginal discharge. Around the ninth month, the discharge becomes heavier and contains more mucus. It may be streaked with blood, (red, pink or brown in color) after a pelvic exam or intercourse.
- Varicose veins in legs. Leg cramps — which may increase

during sleep in the ninth month.
- Increased backache or heaviness.
- Lower abdominal achiness.
- Itchiness of abdomen.
- Protruding naval (around the eighth month).
- Difficulty sleeping.
- Leaking or expressed colostrum from enlarged breasts.
- Increase/decrease in sexual appetite.
- Sporadic Braxton Hicks contractions (the uterus hardens for a minute — then returns to normal). These will increase in the eighth and ninth months, and may be somewhat painful in the ninth month.
- Pelvic or buttock achiness or discomfort toward the eighth–ninth months.
- Increase in need to urinate (usually after the baby drops and puts more pressure on the bladder).

POSSIBLE SIGNS OF MISCARRIAGE

When to call your doctor — just in case:

- If you experience bleeding with cramps or pain in the center of your lower abdomen.
- If pain is severe or continuous — even if it is not accompanied by bleeding.
- If bleeding is heavy (like a menstrual period), or you have light staining for more than three days.

When to obtain emergency medical attention:

- If you have a history of miscarriage, and experience cramping, bleeding or both.
- If you pass clots, grayish, or pinkish material, it may mean that a miscarriage has already begun. If you can't reach your doctor, go immediately to the nearest emergency room. (The doctor may want you to save the material you pass in a plastic bag or other clean container, to help determine if the miscarriage is simply a threat, is incomplete, or complete.

- If bleeding is heavy enough to soak through several pads in an hour, or if pain is severe and/or unbearable.

While waiting for help, lie down if you can, or rest in a chair with your feet up. Although this may not prevent a miscarriage if it is about to happen, it will help you to relax.

Rest assured, however, most women experience some spotting or bleeding in early pregnancy, but carry to term and deliver healthy babies. Mild cramps, achiness, or a pulling sensation on one or both sides of the abdomen is common during pregnancy. This is probably caused by the stretching of ligaments that support the uterus. So there's probably no need to worry unnecessarily.

Nonetheless, tell your doctor about *any* pains, cramping, or bleeding, even if they are mild — just to be on the safe side. Likely, he or she will put your mind at ease.

OTHER REASONS TO CONTACT YOUR PHYSICIAN

The following symptoms may indicate a problem. When you report any of the following, be sure to mention any other symptoms you may have, no matter how unrelated they may seem to be. Be specific. Mention how long the symptom has existed; frequency of occurrence; what exacerbates or seems to relieve it; and how severe the problem(s) is. Call *immediately* for any of the following, except as noted:

- When severe lower abdominal pain does not subside.
- Severe upper, mid–abdominal pain — with or without nausea and swelling of the hands and face.
- Heavy vaginal bleeding — particularly when accompanied with abdominal or back pain. For slight vaginal bleeding, call your physician the same day;
- Coughing up blood.
- A sudden increase in thirst, accompanied by inability to urinate for part or all of the day.
- Bleeding from the nipples, bladder. or rectum — call the same day.
- A gush or consistent leaking of fluid from the vagina.

- Fainting or dizziness.
- If sudden severe swelling or puffiness of hands, face and/or eyes occurs, accompanied by headache or vision difficulty, call immediately. For swelling or puffiness of hands, face or eyes, call the same day.
- Painful or burning sensation while urinating, call practitioner the same day. If accompanied by backache and/or chills and fever over 100 degrees, call immediately.
- Severe headache, persisting for more than two–three hours, call the same day. If accompanied by vision difficulties or puffiness of eyes, face, and/or hands, call immediately.
- Vision disturbances (blurring, double vision, flashes or dimming) persisting for two hours.
- Chills and fever over 100 — in the absence of flu or cold symptoms — call your practitioner immediately.
- Severe nausea and vomiting more than two–three times a day in the first trimester. If you vomit later in pregnancy for no apparent reason, call the same day. If vomiting is accompanied by pain and/or fever, call your doctor immediately.
- Numbness and pain in fingers, call the same day.
- If you have a sudden weight gain of two or more pounds — *not* related to overeating, call the same day. If it accompanied by swelling of the extremities, pain, and/or fever, call immediately.
- All–over itching (with or without dark urine), jaundice (yellowing of the skin), or pale stools, call the same day.
- After the 20th week, if you notice an obvious absence of fetal movement for more than 24 hours, call the same day.

SPECIAL CONCERNS:

DONOR INSEMINATION AND IN–VITRO FERTILIZATION (IVF)

More and more often these days, single women (usually in their mid–to–late thirties) are making the deliberate choice to become mothers. For some, there is no desire to be married or involved in a relationship. For others, biological "time clocks" are running and an appropriate partner is not on the horizon. For many lesbian couples, this is a viable option that makes sense. Whatever the reasons, the trend of donor insemination is steadily growing.

While some may find a donor "candidate" in a friend or lover, others use the services provided at "donor" or "sperm" banks.

What is donor insemination?

Donor, or artificial insemination, is a procedure wherein a sperm donor is used to impregnate a woman. Artificial insemination by donor can be done via Intrauterine Insemination (IUI), or Intravaginal Insemination (IVI).

The IUI method involves injecting sperm into the uterus by means of a catheter directed through the cervix. This method has been practiced for many years. The premise of this procedure is that the sperm can reach and fertilize the egg more easily if they are placed directly into the uterine cavity. The IVI method involves injection of sperm into the vagina in proximity to the cervix rather than into the uterus, as is the case with IUI.

How is a match made?

A donor bank will provide clients with a list of available donors which sets forth the basics, including blood type, ethnic origin, hair color, height and weight, general medical history, family history, educational background and some essay answers. Generally, there is a finite amount of donations one donor can make to a bank. A client will select a donor based upon compatibility and personal preference of donor characteristics.

What is the cost involved in donor insemination?

The cost for this procedure varies. The cost for one day of insemination can range from $50–$80 for a private physician, to $150 at a local hospital's reproductive–endocrine department. Many doctors choose to inseminate two days in a row. In addition to the office visit, the sperm must be purchased. The average rate for a vial of sperm is approximately $135–$165 — and sperm can be frozen or fresh. And the cost for a PCR–HIV test on the sperm is in the range of $175.

The sperm bank will also charge for shipping the sperm. Rates vary but are in the range of $85–$100 — and more than one vial can be shipped at one time. Some banks will ship to your home, while others will only ship to a doctors office.

What is in–vitro fertilization?

In–vitro, or "test tube" fertilization is a technique used primarily in women who are infertile due to diseased, abnormally shaped, or blocked fallopian tubes which cannot be opened by surgery.

In this technique, an egg is removed from the woman's ovary and placed in a test tube or special sterile dish containing the male sperm. Once the egg has been fertilized, it is then placed into the woman's uterus, where it will continue to grow. Although many woman have been successfully impregnated by this method, all forms of female (and male) infertility problems are not treatable by this method.

My baby was conceived through in–vitro fertilization. How is IVF different from other pregnancies?

In the beginning, there will be some differences between an IVF pregnancy and others. Some of the reasons may include: The emotional and financial difficulty of trying again if it doesn't work the first time. Also, a positive test doesn't necessarily mean a pregnancy — which can be very disappointing and emotionally draining. And, there is no way to initially tell how many of the test tube embryos will develop into fetuses.

Additionally, if a mother has miscarried in previous pregnancies, complete bed–rest may be required, and/or intercourse and other activities may be restricted. In some cases, during the first two months, the hormone progesterone may be prescribed to help support the pregnancy. However, once this period passes, IVF pregnancies proceed like a typical pregnancy — unless there is more than one fetus. Approximately 5% – 25% of IVF mothers will carry more than one fetus.

What are my chances of having a normal pregnancy and a healthy baby through IVF?

Recent studies indicate that there is no significant increase in complications such as prematurity, pregnancy–induced hypertension, prolonged labor, need for c–sections, or delivery complications in IVF pregnancies when all other factors (age, condition of uterus, number of fetuses, DES exposure, etc.) are equal. Neither does there appear to be a higher risk of babies being born with abnormalities. However, there is a slightly higher rate of miscarriages. This may be due to the fact that IVF pregnancies are so closely monitored. Therefore, every pregnancy is diagnosed and every miscarriage is detected which is not the case in the general population.

For more information about artificial insemination, talk with your doctor. He or she can refer you to a specialist in the field. Or, contact one of the donor referrals in the Resource Section at the back of this book.

THE AFFECTS OF ALCOHOL, SMOKING, DRUGS AND CAFFEINE ON YOUR FETUS

Alcohol.

Although it was once believed that moderate drinking did not harm or threaten the fetus, it is now believed that alcohol can have devastating effects on the unborn child. Even moderate drinking has been associated with problems. Recent studies indicate that moderate drinking can increase the risk of miscarriage. Other studies associate this level of drinking with more frequent occurrence of birth defects and lower birth weights.

The Food and Drug Administration require that alcoholic beverages carry warning labels to inform pregnant women of the hazards of drinking. And the Surgeon General advises pregnant women (or women considering pregnancy) not to drink alcohol at all.

Studies are inconclusive as to why alcohol is so damaging to an unborn fetus; but they do conclusively show that alcohol affects the brain of the fetus. Babies affected by "fetal alcohol syndrome" are born with physical malformations, including microcephaly (abnormally small head), certain heart defects, and often suffer from mental retardation. It is also known that babies who are born to alcoholics are born addicted to alcohol and often are not normal even after their addiction has been cured.

Because no safe level of alcohol consumption has yet been established for pregnant women, it is advisable to take a cautious approach and refrain from drinking entirely throughout pregnancy.

If you are having trouble stopping your drinking habits during pregnancy, it is advisable to get immediate help or terminate the pregnancy. Contact Alcoholics Anonymous (their number can be found in the white pages) or other sources of assistance in getting sober.

Smoking.

Cigarette smoking poses a serious threat to your unborn child. Mothers who smoke have smaller babies. And there is a greater incidence of miscarriage, prematurity, stillbirth, and death of the baby soon after birth associated with smoking. Babies born to mothers who smoke are also shown to have impaired intellectual and physical development as they grow.

If you can't stop smoking altogether, at the very least, cut down. Try to reduce the number of cigarettes you smoke each day. Take fewer puffs on each cigarette. Cut your cigarettes in half — and smoke only the half with the filter. Choose a brand that is lowest in tar and nicotine. Or, consider entering a program designed to help you quit.

Marijuana.

The question of genetic and metabolic effects of this drug are, as yet, incompletely answered. However, marijuana use has been associated with pulmonary cancer; can cause menstrual irregularities; and is shown to have negative affects on memory.

Studies in animals have shown that the active ingredient in marijuana crosses the placenta and accumulates in the fetus. Effects on the offspring include low–birth weight, intra–uterine growth retardation, and changes in the secondary sex characteristics. Furthermore, in humans, marijuana use is associated with prematurity, prolonged labor, precipitate labor (which ends with rapid expulsion of the baby), arrested labor, greater risk of fetal distress, and low birth weight (though the increased risk is small), among other potential hazards.

Many physicians also feel that use of this and other substances prevent the mother from being in full command of her pregnancy and of the baby after birth — when the baby needs careful attention.

Cocaine/Crack.

Cocaine and crack have very profound effects on the mother and her fetus. They can cause an increase in the mother's heart rate. These substances can cross the placenta (possibly damaging it), and may constrict the blood vessels so that less blood enters the fetus. This can retard fetal growth. It also causes an increase in the secretion of stress hormones which cause constriction of uterine blood vessels, and an increase in uterine contractions.

Cocaine is thought to be associated with a high incidence of spontaneous abortions and placental abruption. And it precipitates a frequent incidence of pregnancy complications, including miscarriage, premature labor, stroke at birth, and stillbirth.

Cocaine or "crack babies" often have abnormal breathing patterns and brain waves. These babies have a very difficult time adjusting to environmental stimuli. And there are numerous other long–term effects, including chronic diarrhea, irritability, excessive crying, developmental delays, and various behavioral problems. Although it is not yet confirmed, it is suspected that these babies are at higher risk of SIDS (sudden infant death syndrome).

Pregnant women who use drugs of any kind — except those prescribed by their physicians, *need to get help!* If you are having problems with drug use or addiction, you are putting your baby at great risk and creating a lifetime of problems for you both. Get professional assistance to help you get off drugs NOW! See the resource section at the end of this book for possible referrals.

Other drugs.

Since no drug has been proved to be safe for the unborn child, and some drugs have been proven to be unsafe, you also need to be cautious about any medications you take. Even over–the–counter remedies can cause problems. Your doctor can help you to decide what, if any, medications are appropriate for you to take during your pregnancy. If you have taken any drugs during your pregnancy, now is the time to discuss this with your physician.

Caffeine.

The most current research on the effects of caffeine on the fetus is inconclusive and less persuasive than those of alcohol or cigarettes. But there is some indication that the equivalent of one and a half to two cups of coffee can double the risk of miscarriage. Until more is known about the possible affects of caffeine and pregnancy, it is prudent to play it safe and refrain from products containing caffeine.

What we do know is that caffeine has a diuretic effect, which may compound the frequent urination that is common with pregnancy. This draws fluid and calcium from the body — both of which are vital to yours and your unborn baby's health. Furthermore, while caffeine (particularly when accompanied by sugar and cream) are filling, they are not nutritious — and may spoil your appetite for the nutritious food you and your child need. Colas, while being "empty" fillers, also contain questionable chemicals and unnecessary sugar.

Research does suggest that excessive caffeine use could result in temporary abnormal heartbeat, rapid respiration, and tremors in newborns — and the development of diabetes. It is suspected that caffeine builds up in the fetal pancreas and eventually damages the cells that produce insulin; though the data is not yet conclusive. In countries where caffeine use is highest, the incidence of diabetes is highest also.

Caffeine may exacerbate your already fluxuating mood swings during pregnancy, and may interfere with your much needed rest. It is also suggested that caffeine may interfere with the absorption of iron by you and your baby.

To help you break the caffeine habit, focus on your baby and his health. Look for substitutes for the caffeine products you use most often — switching to a naturally decaffeinated replacement or a grain beverage from the health food store is helpful. If you drink soft drinks for taste, switch to an occasional caffeine–free cola. Indulge in exercise for the natural boost that caffeine produces artificially.

Though breaking the caffeine habit may be difficult — and you may be edgy or tired for a few days — the benefits to you and your baby will far outweigh your initial discomfort. Though it is best to forego caffeine from the get–go, it is never too late in pregnancy to give it up. Remember, if you're planning to breast–feed, everything you eat goes directly to your baby.

CHAPTER FOUR

TAKING CARE OF YOUR BODY

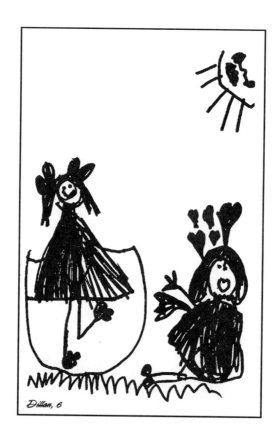

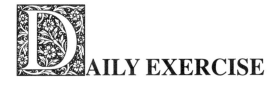

DAILY EXERCISE

Moderate physical activity is considered to be extremely beneficial for most pregnant women and their unborn babies. In fact, if you don't exercise during your pregnancy, you are likely to become progressively less fit as the months pass by and it may be more difficult to lose the extra weight after your baby is born. However, you should *always* consult with your doctor prior to embarking on any exercise routine, even if you are feeling terrific.

If you are healthy and your pregnancy is proceeding normally, once your doctor gives you the go–ahead, you can do most of the same exercises you would do if you were not pregnant.

The benefits of exercise include the following:

- Greater energy, stamina and endurance.
- Strengthens heart muscle; your heart beats fewer times per minute so it rests longer between each beat.
- Increases lung capacity, so there is more oxygen for your blood to distribute to all parts of your body, including your uterus, placenta and your baby.
- Decreases the risk of varicose veins, hemorrhoids, and fluid retention.
- Enhances circulation throughout your entire body. The walls of your blood vessels are toned and strengthened and become more flexible, enabling better circulation.
- Burns calories, allowing you to eat more of the healthy foods you and your baby need without gaining excess weight.
- Psychological benefits. Women who exercise during pregnancy, on average, are likely to feel more calm, relaxed, and refreshed. Exercise also helps to instill a greater sense of happiness and well–being.
- Quicker recovery after birth. Generally women who exercise during pregnancy rebound much faster than those who do not.

Note: **exercise may not be safe under certain conditions.**

If you have heart disease or other chronic ailments — including high blood pressure, anemia, thyroid disease or diabetes — you may need to modify your activities. You may also need to avoid or modify exercise if you have a history of miscarriages, multiple births, bleeding, placenta previa (a condition in which the placenta partially or completely covers the cervix, hindering or preventing vaginal delivery), or an incompetent cervix. If you suffer from any of these conditions, consult with your doctor prior to engaging in any exercise activity or routine — and follow his or her advice.

GUIDELINES OF THE AMERICAN COLLEGE OF OBSTETRICIANS AND GYNECOLOGISTS

The following list covers the basic guidelines (do's and don'ts) of exercising when pregnant:

- Avoid jumping, bouncing, or jerky movements.
- Drink plenty of fluids to prevent dehydration.
- Do not continue strenuous activities for longer than 15 minutes.
- Do not allow your heart rate to exceed 140 beats per minute.
- Do not push yourself too far. Hormone changes during pregnancy increase the looseness of your joints. If you push yourself too hard, you could cause injury.
- Never exercise in hot or humid weather.
- Do not exercise if you are ill or have a fever.
- Exercising should not cause shortness of breath.

In addition to these guidelines, you should not exercise on an empty (or full) stomach. A light snack and drink 15–30 minutes before beginning your warm–ups is advisable. If eating that close to exercising causes you to be uncomfortable, then have your snack an hour before you start.

AVOIDING INJURIES

When exercising, how can I avoid injuries to myself and my baby?

Warm–up exercises. It is very important to do warm–up exercises prior to beginning your routine — especially prior to engaging in more vigorous activities. Spend a minimum of 5–10 minutes stretching and limbering up. Do not stretch to the point where you experience pain. Concentrate first on stretching your lower body (legs, hips, knees and ankles), and then stretch the upper body (neck, shoulders and arms).

A cool down period. Be sure to include a cool–down period after you exercise. Stopping abruptly traps blood in the muscles, reducing blood supply to the other parts of your body and to your fetus. This can cause light–headedness, dizziness, nausea, or extra heartbeats. A cool–down period should consist of gradually slowing down your activity over a period of 5 minutes, and finally stretching your lower and upper body again for 5–10 minutes.

Stick to a routine. Whatever form of exercise you choose, make exercising a routine. Exercising on a regular basis for 20–30 minutes at a time (at least 3 times per week) is preferred over intermittent exercise in order to get the full benefits.

Keep in mind the half–life theory of exercise: if you allow more than 2 days to lapse in between exercising the same muscle group, you will lose the benefit achieved in the first exercise session of those muscles.

Do not take on too much at one time.

Begin with low–intensity exercise activities and gradually build into more advanced routines. You can't make up for lost time, so your routine should gradually increase as you go along. It should not be instantly excessive, especially if you were not exercising prior to your pregnancy.

Never exercise to the point of exhaustion. When you are pregnant, moderation is best. You can begin an exercise regimen during pregnancy even if you did not exercise prior to conception, but you must start out slowly, and only with your doctor's approval and guidance.

Additional precautions.

- Don't point or extend your toes at any time during pregnancy. This can lead to cramping in your calves. Instead, flex feet, turning them upwards toward your upper body.
- Do not stretch to your limit. This can cause damage to joints that have been loosened by pregnancy.
- Don't get up too quickly if you've been exercising on the floor. This can cause dizziness or light–headedness.
- Don't wear socks or tights if the surface is slippery. Avoid surfaces that are uneven. Outdoors, soft, flat, grassy or dirt running areas are better than paved, concrete surfaces. Indoors, tightly carpeted or wood floors are better than concrete or tile for workouts.
- Do not use steam rooms, saunas, hot tubs, or hot baths. These environments are not safe for pregnant women.
- After the fourth month, it is advisable to avoid exercising on your back. The weight of your expanding uterus may compress major blood vessels resulting in restricted circulation.
- Taper off activities during your last three months of pregnancy to avoid injury to you and your fetus — particularly during the final month. Toward the end of your third trimester, stretching routines and brisk walking should provide sufficient exercise.

SIGNS OF TROUBLE DURING EXERCISE

If you experience any pain, discomfort, dizziness, light–headedness, nausea, or extreme fatigue, stop exercising immediately (though it is a good idea to walk around slowly to cool down for a while before sitting down if possible.) These symptoms are warning signs. Listen to your body when it is communicating with you.

If you are experiencing any of these symptoms or other complications, you may need to modify your routine, abandon or substitute certain exercises. In any case, let your doctor know what occurred so that he or she can advise you on resuming your activities.

APPROPRIATE FORMS OF EXERCISE DURING PREGNANCY

What types of exercise can I do?

LOW–IMPACT AEROBIC EXERCISE

Aerobic exercises are rhythmic, repetitive activities which benefit your heart, lungs, and circulatory system (your cardiopulmonary system). They also stimulate muscle and joint activity. Appropriate forms of aerobic exercise during pregnancy include: stretching, walking, stepping, swimming, bicycling (with extreme caution), rowing, and dancing. Some doctors will allow their patients to run if they engaged in this activity prior to pregnancy. But be sure you consult with your doctor before you engage in running exercise.

CALISTHENICS

Calisthenics are rhythmic, light gymnastic movements which will help to tone and develop muscles. However, you should only engage in calisthenics designed especially for pregnant women. Calisthenics can help to relieve back pain, improve posture, and enhance your physical and mental well–being.

KEGEL EXERCISE

Kegel exercise is a simple technique. Kegel's tone and tighten your pelvic floor muscles in the vaginal and perineal area, preparing you for childbirth. To help you discover the muscle group, try stopping the flow of urine midstream by tightening the muscles. However, unless you need to find the muscle group again, discontinue the practice while urinating.

Once you discover the muscle group, you can then do Kegel's in virtually any position; sitting, standing or lying down in a comfortable position. Twenty to thirty sets of Kegel's per day is recommended for maximum benefit. Because these muscles fatigue easily, a set should consist of three to five squeezes at a time intermittently throughout the day. When squeezing, hold tightly for a count of two or three and release; repeat. *Note:* if you are standing, the farther apart you position your legs, the more challenging this exercise will be.

WALKING – A GOOD PLACE TO START

If you are not already in the practice of daily or semi–weekly exercise, a good place for you to start is with walking. If you are out of shape, walking is terrific because you can start out at your own pace. Walk at a slow pace to the corner first, then build up to a walk around the block — gradually increasing the pace and the distance.

Ultimately, a reasonable goal would be to walk in the range of a mile and a half to two and a half miles (depending upon your level of fitness) in 20 minutes or so. Walking is excellent for your cardiovascular system, for weight maintenance, for body tone, and for peace of mind.

Mornings – a time to reflect.

During my second pregnancy, I took the opportunity to walk first thing in the morning before I left my house for work. I took that time to be quiet and reflective and to enjoy the natural surroundings outdoors. Sometimes I listened to music, but more often I did what I call "walking meditation".

I would focus on the beauty of nature; the flowers, trees, birds, sunshine and fresh air; and would talk and sing quietly to my unborn baby (people driving by must have thought I was nuts!) I took time on those walks to repeat positive affirmations; to clear my head of all negative or uninvited thoughts; and to focus upon good and positive images. I planned for my baby's arrival and imagined what my life would be like when he was born.

When I felt at odds with the world; with my baby's father; my hormones; or whatever, those walks turned me right around and gave me the energy I needed to face the day. I found mornings to be the best time of day to get out and walk because they helped to kick–start my day. It was a great time bond with my unborn baby and the pollution levels from car exhaust were at their lowest levels.

What types of exercise should I avoid during pregnancy?

- Jogging more than two miles per day, unless your doctor approves.
- Horseback riding.
- Waterskiing.
- Scuba diving (diving gear can restrict circulation, and decompression sickness is hazardous to the baby).
- Diving and jumping into swimming pools.
- Downhill skiing (a fall could be very risky to your fetus).
- Cross–country skiing above 10,000 feet. The high altitude will deprive both you and your fetus of oxygen.
- Sprinting. Too much oxygen is required too quickly.
- Contact sports, such a basketball or football.
- Calisthenics not specifically designed for pregnancy, including (but not limited to) full sit–ups or double leg lifts which will pull on the abdomen; jerky, bouncy, jumping motions; contortions that involve deep flexation or extension of joints (such as deep knee bends).

GETTING MOTIVATED!

Sometimes I just don't feel like exercising.

There may be some days when you just don't feel like getting out of bed, let alone doing exercises. You may be tempted to pass on your usual routine. If you indulge yourself here or there, that's fine. Just don't make a habit of it.

You need to get motivated! Think about your health, and the health of your unborn baby. Both you and your baby need the benefits of exercise. When you're not in the mood for a workout, you'll likely find if you push yourself to do it anyway, you will feel much better physically and emotionally.

Give yourself reinforcement. Send positive messages to your brain: "I can do this!" If it inspires you, play music on a Walkman. Turn the radio up on your stereo and dance around the house. Get a buddy to join you in your workout, or join a prenatal exercise class.

Prenatal exercise classes and videos.

As your second trimester progresses, you may want to consider joining a specially designed prenatal exercise class. Or get your hands on one of the many terrific prenatal videos available on the market.

Prenatal exercise classes and videos are designed to help you gain maximum benefit from exercise while helping you avoid unnecessary stress or strain on your body. Check with your health club, local YWCA, college, community center, or department of parks and recreation to see if they offer such a program.

Wear appropriate clothing when exercising.

Your clothing should be loose–fitting and comfortable. If you are engaging in aerobic exercise, walking, or running, it would be wise to invest in a good pair of shoes which provide lateral support, cushioning, traction and flexibility. These features are very important for your safety as well as for your comfort.

A good support bra is also important. You will find that your breasts become larger and more tender both during your pregnancy and after if you are breast-feeding. So be sure that any bra you select provides you with adequate support; that it is well made; and that it fits you comfortably. If you are nursing, wearing a nursing bra beneath a sports bra may work very well for you and provide you with additional support.

CHECKING YOUR VITAL SIGNS DURING EXERCISE

Monitoring your pulse.

You will want to monitor your pulse while working out. Try to keep moving while you check your pulse because if you stop and stand still to check it, your pulse will drop or change and you won't get an accurate reading.

To count your pulse, place your index and middle fingers of your right hand on your left wrist. When you locate your pulse beat, begin counting how many times you feel the beat during six second intervals. You will count the first beat as zero, followed by one, two, three, four, five, and so on. You then add a zero to the number you count (i.e., if you count thirteen beats, your pulse would be 130).

You may find you need to practice monitoring your pulse to become good at it. But it is very important for you to do so to make sure that your pulse is in the right range, so continue to practice.

Determining your heart rate zone.

In order to receive the benefits of exercise and to improve your heart muscle, it is important that you keep your pulse within your target heart rate zone. During your pregnancy and for approximately twelve weeks after delivery, your target heart rate zone is achieved when your heart is beating at between 60–70% of your safe maximum attainable heart rate.

The formula which is used to determine each person's individual target zone is as follows: 220 (which is considered the highest pulse) minus your age equals your safe maximum attainable heart rate. Multiply that number by 60 and 70% to get the limits of your target zone. For example: $220 - 35 = 185 \times 60\%/70\% = 111-129.50$.

Use your target zone to help you regulate your activity during exercise. If your pulse is below your target zone, you need to increase your activity. If it is above your target zone, you need to slow it down.

The following chart is broken down by age to help you determine your target zone:

AGE	TARGET HEART RATE ZONE (in beats per minute)
20	120–140
21	119–139
22	118–138
23–24	117–137
25	116–136
26–27	115–135
28	114–134
29–30	113–133
31	112–132
32	111–131
33–34	110–130
35	109–129
36–37	108–128
38	107–127
39–40	106–126
41	105–125
42	104–124

Note: Target heart rate zone for pregnant and postpartum women is calculated at sixty percent of the safe maximum attainable heart rate. In pregnancy, maximum heart rate should never exceed 140 beats per minute.

Endorphins: A boost to physical and mental well–being

Besides the obvious physical health benefits gained by you and your unborn baby as a result of exercise, your body creates endorphins (a naturally produced opiate–like substance), which are secreted into the brain causing what some describe as a "natural high".

The chemical reaction of the endorphins creates a surge of energy which causes us to feel more upbeat and energized. The benefits of a higher level of energy is obvious, particularly when the stress of pregnancy takes its toll upon our bodies and emotions. The result is that this higher level of energy creates emotional well–being – which in turn encourages us to continue the exercise that improves our physical conditioning.

EATING HEALTHY

It's always important to eat a well–rounded, nutritious, calorie and fat–conscious diet, especially when you are pregnant. Your diet before and during your pregnancy provides the essential nutrients needed for your baby's development and healthy growth. Because the fetus derives all of its nutrition directly from the mother, it is essential that a well–rounded diet is maintained.

In attempting to maintain the healthiest diet possible, now is a good time to consider eating organically grown foods. Unfortunately, many of the vegetables, fruits, dairy, and other products sold in regular grocery stores are treated with pesticides and contain hormones which can harm you, your fetus, and your growing child. Though organically grown products may cost more, many doctors believe they are a lot healthier for human consumption — particularly for your fetus and small children. You may want to investigate alternative food sources both during and after pregnancy.

What impact do my eating habits have on my unborn child?

Your baby is formed from the nutritional elements – good or bad – consumed by you. At first, the fetus is nourished from the yolk sac. As it develops, it draws nutrients directly from your blood stream through the placenta and the umbilical cord.

The foods you eat will directly influence the development of your baby's heart, lungs, bones and brain. Thus, it is essential that you watch what and how you are eating. If your intake is low in certain nutrients, it is likely that your baby will "feed" upon whatever nutrients are available before you absorb your required nutrients, thus depleting your reserves. This can cause serious problems in your health, and jeopardize your baby's health and growth as well.

Malnutrition, among pregnant women is often the cause of low–birth–weights in infants. These are the babies who are statistically most likely to suffer from a variety of medical problems or complications. Some of these complications could have been avoided if the dietary habits of the mother were more aligned with her and her baby's needs.

Doctors and nutritionists commonly agree that a proper diet in pregnant women results in a reduction of health problems and mortality in newborns. Eating well during your pregnancy to meet the increased nutritional demands of your body will not only benefit the baby, it will also contribute to a healthier pregnancy for you.

Special eating concerns.

Under the following circumstances, *always* talk to your doctor about your dietary needs — preferably at your first prenatal exam:

If you are a vegetarian, or avoid certain major food group(s), you will need to take extra care to supplement the missing food group with the proper, equivalent food groups.

If you are anemic, on a special diet for a medical condition, or suffer from an eating disorder (such as bulimia or anorexia), in these cases, it is particularly important to take extra care to make sure you receive proper nutrition. A nutritionist can be very helpful in formulating a healthy prenatal diet especially for you. Ask your doctor for a referral.

I haven't been too careful about what I've been eating so far. Is it too late to change my eating habits?

It is never too late to pay attention to what you are eating. If you have maintained poor eating habits up to this point, *now* is definitely the time to change those habits!

Ideally, nutrition for your fetus begins even before you become pregnant. Because the foods you eat determine your stores of calcium, iron and other nutrients important to your fetus's development, if you have not yet done so, changing your habits now is better than never changing them at all. In doing so, you will minimize the risks of giving birth to an unhealthy child.

Of course, the better the quality of food you eat, the better you will feel. If you are over–indulging in fast food, sugar, fatty foods, overly processed food, etc., it will most assuredly have an affect on your state of mind as well as the quality of your pregnancy and delivery. An occasional indulgence in a great hamburger or other type of "junk food" is not going to hurt you or your fetus. But keeping to a healthful, well–balanced diet consisting of nutritional, high quality foods will clearly benefit you both.

PRENATAL VITAMIN SUPPLEMENTS

Adequate nourishment, and prenatal supplemental vitamins and minerals, are essential to building new tissues in the fetus. They are also necessary to replenish cells in your body that are being drained by the new life growing within you.

It is difficult to maintain a nutritionally perfect diet everyday during pregnancy, particularly in the early weeks when morning sickness may suppress your appetite — and vomiting may deplete the nutritional benefit of the food that won't stay down.

While a good prenatal vitamin will not replace a good prenatal diet, it will help. Some studies have shown that women who take prenatal vitamins prior to pregnancy and during the first month significantly reduce the risk of neural tube defects (such as spina bifida) in their babies.

Your doctor will prescribe a prenatal vitamin. Do not take any other kind of dietary supplement without your physician's recommendation. If you have side effects from your vitamin — such as increased nausea, constipation or diarrhea, consult with your doctor. He or she can advise you about switching supplements. Never switch prenatal vitamin supplements without first consulting your doctor.

NAUSEA

If nausea, commonly referred to as morning sickness, occurs in the first trimester of your pregnancy, it can temporarily affect your weight gain and make for some pretty rough moments. This condition usually disappears by the fourth month of pregnancy.

If you are troubled by morning sickness (which, by the way, does not only occur in the morning), try eating three or four dry crackers with a half a glass of milk. Keep the crackers handy if you experience nausea throughout your day. They should help to settle your stomach.

Until the nausea subsides, keep your meals simple and small, and avoid coffee, tea, high–fat, greasy, fried and spicy foods. Also, avoid strong odors which may bother you and cause nausea.

Because your stomach will shrink in size as the baby grows, your stomach's capacity to hold food decreases. It will probably be more comfortable for you to eat several smaller meals throughout the day instead of three typically large meals.

DAILY CALORIC INTAKE
AND WEIGHT GAIN DURING PREGNANCY

I Feel so fat! Can I diet while I am pregnant?

No! As your doctor will tell you, never attempt to diet while you are pregnant. Dieting can be harmful to your growing fetus. However, you will want to pay attention to your caloric intake in order to watch your overall weight gain.

If you are feeling fat, or unattractive as a result of your ever expanding figure, it will be very helpful if you learn to get over being self–conscious early on. Lamenting about every pound you gain will unnecessarily make things harder on you. Instead of focusing on how you look, concentrate on how you feel. There's a beautiful little baby growing inside of you — so of course you're going to get bigger and bigger! Appreciate the beauty, the miracle, and the elegance of being pregnant.

Is it possible to gain too much weight during pregnancy?

Yes. Excessive weight gain can cause unnecessary problems for you and your baby. Additionally, extra weight will be much more difficult to get rid of once your baby is born. And it will cause the road back to your pre–pregnancy weight to be more of an uphill climb than it really has to be.

During my first pregnancy, I did not pay attention to the important role of nutrition on my pregnancy. Thus, by the eighth month, I had gained 57 (count em') 57 pounds! Not at all healthy or reasonable.

Although I felt great during my first pregnancy, at eight months I had become bloated and developed pre–eclampsia (elevated blood pressure, swelling, and kidney malfunction). The doctors had to induce labor early because of the condition. If I had been more aware of my diet and its effect on my pregnancy, the pre–eclampsia would likely have been avoided.

During my second pregnancy, I was more conscientious about weight gain. I was determined to restrict my weight gain to a more reasonable and healthy amount. I paid close attention to the foods I ate, and remained healthy during my pregnancy — gaining a healthy 27 pounds. I felt and looked terrific, and I had no complications with the pregnancy.

Recommended weight gain.

The recommended daily caloric intake during pregnancy is approximately 2,100 to 2,400 calories. Your weight gain during pregnancy should be slight in the first trimester, with more rapid weight gain during the second and third trimester. Toward the end of your pregnancy, due to the demands of your growing fetus, your body may require more energy from the foods it burns.

It is possible that your caloric intake may rise to as high as 2600 calories per day during the later part of your pregnancy. However, if you are not as active as you were earlier in your pregnancy, your caloric intake may not need to increase.

There will be a wide–range in weight gain and pattern of weight gain during pregnancy from one woman to another. The following averages are simply a guide. You may find that your weight gain does not follow these guidelines. Throughout your pregnancy, your doctor will monitor your weight gain and instruct you accordingly.

The average weight gain during pregnancy is between 25–35 pounds, depending upon your pre–pregnancy size and weight. If you are underweight, petite or small boned to begin with, you will likely be advised to gain closer to 30 pounds. If you are of normal, or average weight, a weight gain of between 25–30 pounds will be appropriate. If you are overweight (weighing more than 35% above the ideal body weight), your doctor will likely urge you to gain between 15–25 pounds. Because these are average figures, you should rely upon your doctor's advice to determine the appropriate weight gain for your height and body weight.

WEIGHT GAIN DISTRIBUTION DURING PREGNANCY

	(Average) Weight
The baby	7.5
The amniotic fluid	1.8
The placenta	1.4
Increase in uterus's weight	2.1
Increase in mother's blood	2.7
Increase in breasts' weight	0.9
Additional fluid	3.7
Increase in mother's fat stores	4.0–8.0
Total (approximate) weight gain	24.1–28.1 pounds

MEETING YOUR NUTRITIONAL NEEDS

The following guide will help you to decide if your dietary intake is sufficient for your pregnancy. Pay attention to the serving size and variety within these food groups:

FOOD CATEGORY	PRIMARY NUTRIENTS OR NUTRITIONAL BENEFITS	NUMBER OF RECOMMENDED DAILY SERVINGS	EXAMPLES OF SINGLE SERVINGS
DAIRY	Calcium phosphorus, vitamin D, protein	4	8oz. milk, 1-1/2 oz. cheese, 1-1/3 cups cottage cheese, 1-1/2 cups ice cream
HIGH QUALITY PROTEIN	Complete protein, iron, folate, vitamin A, B-complex vitamins	3-4	2-3 oz. meat, 2 medium eggs, 1 cup tofu, 1 cup baked beans, 1 cup dried peas, 1/2 cup nuts, 1/4 cup peanut butter
GRAINS AND BREADS	B-complex vitamins, iron, incomplete proteins, (also provide fiber and energy)	4 or more (as needed for for calories)	1 slice bread (enriched or wholegrain), 1/2 cup brown rice, 1/2 cup macaroni, 1/2 cup cooked cereal, 1 tortilla or bagel, 1 tbsp. wheat germ
GREEN AND YELLOW VEGATABLES	Vitamin A, folate, vitamin E, vitamin C, riborflavin, magnesium, iron	1-2	1/2 cup spinach, 3/4 cup carrots, 1 sm. stalk broccoli, 1 sm. sweet potato, 3-1/2 oz. romaine lettuce, 1/2 cup squash
CITRUS FRUITS, FRUITS AND VEGETABLES RICH IN VITAMIN C	Vitamin C, folate	1-2	1 orange or 1/2 cup orange juice, 1/2 cup grapefruit, 1 cup tomato juice or 1 large tomato, 3/4-cup strawberries, 3/4 cup cabbage, 1/2 green pepper
POTATOES AND OTHER FRUITS AND VEGETABLES	Vitamins (also provides fiber and energy)	1 or more as needed for calories	1 potato, 1/2 cup corn, 1/2 cupcauliflower, 1/2 cup celery, 1/2 cup beets, 1/2 cup eggplant
FATS	Vitamin A, vitamin E (also provide energy)	1-2	1 tbsp. butter, margarine, oil, mayonnaise, or salad dressing

FOOD CATEGORY	PRIMARY NUTRIENTS OR NUTRITIONAL BENEFITS	NUMBER OF RECOMMENDED DAILY SERVINGS	EXAMPLES OF SINGLE SERVINGS
LIQUIDS	Required due to increased metabolic rate (will also increase comfort)	2-3 quarts (and as needed to satisfy thirst)	1 8oz. glass water, juice or other beverage (avoid alcohol and caffeine)
IODINE CONTAINING FOODS	Iodine	salt to taste	Iodized salt (in moderation), seafood
FOODS CONSISTING PRIMARILY OF NON-NUTRITIOUS CALORIES	(Provide energy)	eat in mod-moderation only after daily nutritional needs have been met	Sugar, candy bar, cookies, jam, syrup, honey

During your pregnancy, it is recommended that you cut out excess sugar and fat as much as is possible from your diet. You should use salt in moderation (studies indicate that salt is a necessary ingredient in a pregnant woman's diet.) If you are in good health and your pregnancy is progressing normally, you will not need to change your other seasoning habits.

Drink plenty of liquids, including lots of water during your pregnancy (and after). You should not include alcohol as part of your liquid intake, as it is potentially harmful to your fetus.

To be or not to be Betty Crocker...

For some people, cooking will be more of a chore than it is a pleasure. It may be that you simply do not like to cook, or it may be that "he's" not there to cook for, or to enjoy a meal with you. Whatever your reasons, if you have a kitchen "phobia", during pregnancy, it is not the time to indulge in it. Now, more than ever you need to take a good look at the foods you are preparing (or not preparing) and eating.

It may be tempting (and far easier) for you to eat take–out or fast foods, or to rely on frozen dinners during your pregnancy. You need to be very careful in this area, because take–out foods and many frozen foods are often most high in fat, grease and salt. You need to make the extra effort to eat healthy meals.

To conserve, and more effectively manage your time, you can prepare meals large enough to freeze and store portions for future use. Perhaps you'll never be a kitchen whiz (and maybe you don't want to be). But with very little effort, you can prepare easy, simple, and yet nutritional meals. Get your hands on charts and books to show you, quick, tasteful recipes. Be creative and remember your goal: having a healthy pregnancy and baby.

After your baby's birth, if you plan to breast–feed, see Chapter Seven, *Feeding – Breast or Bottle*, page 122 for more information on breast–feeding and your diet.

REST AND SLEEP DURING PREGNANCY

You are apt to be more tired or easily fatigued when you are pregnant due to the increasing needs of the baby growing within you, so it is likely to take you longer to regain your energy level. That's why it is especially important during your pregnancy to get enough rest and sleep. Usually eight to ten hours of sleep at night, and a rest during the day, should be sufficient to maintain your energy level. Needs will vary from woman to woman, so listen to your body and follow what it tells you.

I'm working and I'm so tired — help! — what's going on?

If you are working during your pregnancy, it is especially important for you to notice, and yield to the signs your body is giving you. You will probably be more tired than usual during the first few months. In fact, it would be surprising if you weren't. Activities that did not cause fatigue before your pregnancy now create exhaustion.

During the first trimester of your pregnancy, your body is hard at work developing the placenta (your baby's life support system). This activity can really zap your energy! Additionally, the other physical and emotional demands of your pregnancy may also be taking their toll.

As your pregnancy progresses, your job and other responsibilities, along with the extra weight you are now carrying, will deplete your energy. During this period you may also be losing sleep at night. With your expanding waist line making it difficult to find a comfortable position, and other distractions crowding your mind, you may find sleeping at night harder than it was before.

GETTING ADEQUATE REST

Throughout both of my pregnancies, I often went down to my car to take a nap during my lunch hour. It made a remarkable difference in my level of energy and ability to continue my work throughout the rest of the day. If you can slip away during your lunch hour to close your eyes and rest — even if only for 15–20 minutes — you will likely feel rejuvenated. A short, 5 minute meditation at your desk can also help (see Chapter Six, page 82, for more information on the benefits of meditation).

You may need more or less sleep at different times. You may find you need to go to sleep at night earlier. Become aware and flexible about your body's demands and needs. Your body will tell you when you need to draw back the reins and slow down.

The more quickly you respond to fatigue by beginning to rest, the more quickly your body will get rid of the metabolic waste products that caused you to be fatigued in the first place. As you rest, your body will activate new energy reserves.

You may have a reprieve during your second trimester (around the fourth month). After your body has adjusted to your pregnancy, you will probably have more energy. However, you may feel extremely fatigued again in your last trimester (around the seventh month) — though some women have intermittent bursts of energy around the ninth month.

Adequate rest will benefit your unborn baby.

When you are asleep, you have what are called rapid eye movements (REM) during the various sleep cycles. REM sleep is associated with high levels of growth hormones. Such hormones penetrate the placenta and reach the baby. Growth hormones are believed to stimulate brain growth in the baby.

In contrast, when you are fatigued/stressed, these hormones reach the baby as well. If you keep this in mind, and act accordingly to get adequate rest and sleep, your baby and you will both benefit.

Don't take on too much at one time.

Since you will likely be mostly dependent upon yourself to do your daily chores (grocery shopping, laundry, house cleaning, etc.), you will need to make sure you do not take on too much at one time. Take naps if you can, especially on weekends. If you are feeling tired, slow down on unnecessary activities. It's also a good idea to enlist friends or neighbors to help you out when they can, especially with heavy jobs or heavy lifting – which can harm your unborn baby.

CHAPTER FIVE

YOUR MOODS AND FEELINGS

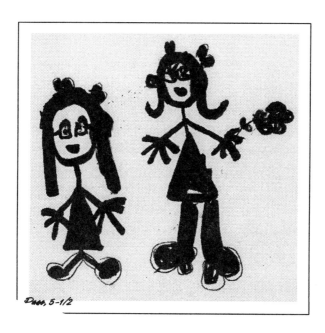

Dee, 5-1/2

N ARRAY OF EMOTIONS

Your feelings are the reactions, pleasurable or unpleasur-able, that you have to the various situations in your life. They are not based in logic. They come from your perception or conception of the people, places and things around you. Because they originate in your mind, they are subjective and cannot be judged. In other words, feelings are not right or wrong. But they cause a variety of moods within you.

Every person is entitled, and indeed expected, to have an array of moods — particularly pregnant women! Depression, anger, frustration, resentments, fear, sadness, loneliness, laziness, over–sensitivity, insensitivity to others, irritability, childishness, happiness, glee, love, generosity, nostalgia, vibrancy, charm, among others, are all a part of us at one time or another.

Unlike characteristics or personality traits, moods are never fixed and seldom can be accurately defined or correlated with particular "types" of people. A spectrum of moods is inherent in all of us. And they continue to change as we respond to a variety of different feelings, stimulation, life events, etc. While you can sometimes exert a certain amount of control over your moods, they just are what they are.

Help! Since my pregnancy began, I feel like I'm out of control.

During your pregnancy, you are apt to experience feelings and emotions which swing from one end of the spectrum to the other. The increased physical demands on your body, your hormones, and the normal expectations and fears of your pregnancy, often cause you to feel like you're on a roller coaster. One moment you're elated, powerful and optimistic. The next moment, you burst into tears and doubt your abilities to do this. Mood swings may fluxuate so widely that you wonder if you are going nuts. The fact that you are doing this without a partner to nurture you may add to your distress and can make life seem even harder.

Your moods and feelings will probably be exaggerated throughout pregnancy. Small incidents may seem like monumental events, as sensitivity is heightened. A pregnant woman may cry if somebody appears to look at her the wrong way. She may be edgy over matters that usually do not concern her. Or, in the case of a single pregnancy, she may be angry over her "aloneness." Any number of emotions may come up. For many of us, that's just the way it is.

If you (or somebody else) thinks you're being silly, foolish or overreacting, remember that your moods and feelings belong to you and are valid. There are no "proper" or "correct" feelings about your situation. What you feel is what you feel. But do keep in mind that your underlying beliefs about certain things will have an impact on your feelings and in turn, will ultimately affect your moods.

If you find that your mood swings are severe; if you are feeling seriously depressed for any length of time; or you are acting out in inappropriate ways, it is advisable to seek professional help.

I want more raisins!!!

One morning during my second pregnancy, I met some friends at a restaurant for breakfast. With my eggs and toast, I ordered some milk and Raisin Bran. When I opened the single size serving box of cereal and out poured two raisins, (count em' two!) I was devastated. The friends who were with me thought it was funny. I didn't think it was so funny at all; I wanted "two scoops of raisins" in my morning cereal! Normally, I would consider such an experience uneventful, but because I was hormonal (i.e., pregnant) and very hungry, I was upset.

In this situation, I may have expressed "silly" emotions. I may have even overreacted, but I felt better about having a good cry over it than I would have if I had stuffed my feelings. Ultimately, I wrote a letter to the company, (good self–assertive practice), and they responded with an apology and coupon for a free box of cereal.

I am sharing this incident to point out that most pregnant women are extremely sensitive. We can react to the strangest situations in very emotional ways. At times we may be reacting to very dramatic or serious difficulties. Other times we may over–react to those "silly" little things that go on around us day–to–day.

Have a good cry if it helps — howl at the moon!

When mood swings occur, simply allow yourself to feel, experience and express your emotions. Bottling them up and pretending they do not exist is not healthy for you or your unborn child.

There are many times when it is best to let go, get it out, and clear the air. Have a good cry if it helps. Hit your pillow if you are angry. Howl at the moon. Write a letter. Allow yourself to feel your emotions. Don't be too proud to ask a friend to listen, and don't pretend you're in such control or so strong that you don't have feelings. It's okay to be human.

Some of the emotions you may encounter during your pregnancy include:

DEPRESSION

I feel so depressed. What's wrong with me? Shouldn't I be happy during my pregnancy?

Is it possible that you are mistaking depression for the normal mood swings of pregnancy? If you suffered from emotional instability premenstrually, your mood swings may be more pronounced during the first few months of pregnancy. And feelings of fear, ambivalence, etc., about your pregnancy — or the loss of a partner — may exaggerate your moods even more.

If, however, you find that you are consistently or frequently depressed, you might be one of the 10% of women who battle against mild–to–moderate depression during pregnancy. Some factors which can contribute to such depression include:

- Lack of support from your baby's father and others.
- A history of personal or family mood disorders.
- Money worries.
- Complications of pregnancy; doctor–ordered bed rest; or hospitalization.
- Worries over your baby's, or your own health — particularly if you've had complications with a previous pregnancy, or history of miscarriage.
- Work–related stress or lack of sleep.
- Improper diet.

If you're experiencing sleep disturbances, prolonged or unusual fatigue, lethargy, increase/decrease in eating habits, or exaggerated mood swings, speak to your physician about your depression — or ask for a referral to a therapist.

LONELINESS

Whether you are independent and accustomed to living by yourself, or you are newly on your own after having lived with someone for a period of time, loneliness is a common feeling experienced by many women — particularly pregnant women. However, the degree to which a woman may experience loneliness will vary.

While some women will not experience loneliness at all, others will experience loneliness as periodic bouts of the "blues" or slight depression. Still others may experience a more pronounced, profound sense of loneliness, isolation or depression. Your experience will be unique to you and your circumstances.

Throughout your pregnancy, you may find yourself longing for the comfort of having your ex–lover or husband at your side, or for male companionship in your life. Feeling frustrated at not being able to share the various landmarks or excitement of your pregnancy and childbirth with someone special can also be very depressing. Right now you may be feeling like it would be very soothing to be with someone whom you love.

If you are experiencing feelings of loneliness, rest assured that they are natural and normal. In fact, it's not a secret that many married or coupled women experience loneliness within their relationships. Indeed, many married women feel "single." Having a man in your life doesn't necessarily guarantee that you will not experience some degree of emptiness. But when you are pregnant, being with someone can look pretty good. Nonetheless, you can do certain things for yourself to help to diminish or quiet those feelings of loneliness or isolation.

Allow your friends and family to comfort you and to care for you. Ask a friend if you can call in the middle of the night if you get lonely. Perhaps you are a member of a church or a group of some sort which can support you through these times. Get out and do things.

Be good to yourself. Take action when possible to help yourself through these rough spots. This may sound easier said than done; but if you do not take care of yourself and take steps to help you through these emotions, the feelings will surely stay the same or get worse.

There also may be times when nothing and nobody can soothe your feelings of loneliness. These are the times that you need to hold on tight and walk through your feelings one moment at a time. In these instances, you may want to try some of the exercises in this book (meditation, writing, etc.) to help you to pull it back together. Accepting that your hormones are raging, that you are doing this pregnancy on your own, and that loneliness is a part of it, will also be very important for you.

FRUSTRATION

We become frustrated when we are let–down, disappointed, or feel that our efforts are in vain — or not creating the results we want.

For many pregnant women, as the months progress and the abdomen expands, frustration becomes an increasing emotion. The limitations that go along with pregnancy can begin to feel as if they are closing in around us, giving us the feeling that we'll never get back to normal.

For me, it was frustration that I couldn't wear my 501 Levis. I felt that if I ever saw another pair of stretchy pants again, I would scream. For Kathleen, it was frustration over her difficulty sleeping comfortably after her fifth month. Janet found her boyfriend's failure to follow through on his promises to be there for her during her pregnancy extremely frustrating and hurtful.

Whatever the scenario, our level of frustration is often intensified during pregnancy. Being aware that this heightened sense of frustration is temporary, will help.

ANGER

Anger arises from feelings of displeasure or resentment resulting from perceived injury or mistreatment by another. Often this feeling causes us to feel like fighting back at the supposed cause of the problem. But fighting back is usually more destructive than constructive. While a certain amount of anger over certain situations is normal and healthy, what we do about our anger is another matter.

If your goal is a happy, healthy pregnancy — which I'm sure it is — you will want to avoid situations and/or people that stir up this emotion. Nonetheless, you may feel angry at times — particularly when you are experiencing fear.

When this occurs, expressing your anger in a constructive manner is the best way to resolve your conflict. If you are angry over a particular situation, you shouldn't be expected to be a doormat and sit silently by as you accept mistreatment or abuse. Instead, identify the problem and then take rational, constructive steps to talk about it in an effort to resolve the conflict. Going into "attack" mode will hardly ever correct the problem. And defensiveness begets defensiveness.

RESENTMENTS

Resentments occur when we are unwilling or unable to let go of our anger or frustrations. This anger or frustration, which precipitates resentments, causes us to feel deprived and deeply bitter. But the problem is, this emotion subtly — or obviously — eats away at our ability to experience personal joy and freedom.

Resentments may be a big issue for you. You may feel bitter about any number of things. The "system" that failed you; the difficulty of being on your own; or a job where you are underpaid or under–appreciated. For many of you, the resentments you have toward your ex — particularly if he left you and your child to fend for yourselves — will be a *BIG* issue. But even when these feelings are justified, they need to be resolved and healed.

A sack of emotions.

Imagine that your anger or resentments are carried in a very large, heavy and burdensome sack on your back. This sack contains the weight of each of your negative emotions and feelings. The more negative the emotions, the heavier the sack is for you to carry.

If you continue to carry this extra load, ultimately you will find that the extra weight of those resentments hurt and hinder you more than they do the person or thing to whom they are directed. Thus, each day as you walk through your life, unless you take action to lighten your load, you are unnecessarily burdened by the extra weight of the weight of the sack.

However, when you take responsibility for your feelings as they arise, and practice letting go of negativity (by using the ideas in this book and others), you will be able to release one, then another, of these emotions. The sack will gradually become lighter and more easily carried.

You will soon find that you are not weighed down by so many troubles, and your baby will not be burdened with them either. Keep in mind that our children inherit our sack as they grow! This is part of our legacy to them.

As you travel the road of pregnancy and parenting, I hope that you will keep this in mind and take steps to remove those barriers from your path so that your heart and mind will open up to more freedom, compassion, joy and love. Keep in mind that if you don't release negative energies, they will surely cause you to be unhappy and even physically ill.

I'm not sure I'm able, or willing to let go of certain resentments.

Clearly, some resentments will be easier to let go of than others. Some may even seem impossible to be rid of.

I know from experience that resentments can be the most difficult of feelings to overcome. But they are on the top of the "most important things to discard" list. Particularly when you consider that your resentments will influence your future relationships, choices, and decisions. With this in mind, the question to ask yourself is: "Do I really want to experience peace in my life?"

Your willingness to let go of these burdens will go a long way toward helping to prompt you to take action to release them. Once you are willing to stop blaming others and move on to find solutions to help you get free of such negative burdens, you will find peace. But this is a process that requires action on your part.

If you are not willing to let go of your anger or resentments, be assured that your unwillingness will stand in the way of a healing process. So get ready and get willing! Whether you're feeling troubled or wonderful, writing is an effective tool.

FEAR

Fear is the general term for the anxiety and agitation felt at the presence of danger. But the question we would do well to ask ourselves is, how much of the day–to–day fear we experience as human beings is the result of *real* danger vs. *imagined* danger?

So many of us walk through life "manufacturing" fear which then blocks us from experiencing happiness. This fear of our own creation always distorts our perception and confuses us about what is really going on in our lives. So, ask yourself this question: "What causes me fear?' And then take a look at your answers.

Are these fear–based feelings of anxiety, dread, apprehension and pain about *real* dangers, or are they creations of your mind? Observe how they inhibit your willingness to stretch your boundaries, try again, take risks, challenge authority, and grow beyond mediocrity.

I'm not saying that a certain amount of fear isn't appropriate or necessary. In many cases fear serves an important purpose. It can protect us from certain dangers, for example walking through a dark alley alone late at night. However, much of our fear is not about *real* dangers — and it causes us to be unnecessarily paralyzed.

This manufactured fear can be so great that we stay "stuck" in situations that are unhealthy and unhappy for us. After all, the unknown is often more frightening than what we already know. Whether it's a bad relationship, an unfulfilling job, fear of going back to school, or fear of displeasing someone, we often forsake growth and change because we are afraid to risk.

As a single mother, if I stayed too long in fear–based thought modes, I would not be very happy — because many of the challenges I face are initially fearful to me. But I decided early on not to let my fear get the best of me.

To help me overcome my fears, I have found it useful to separate the *real* from the *imagined*. And I take action in any case to walk through whatever challenge is presented — one foot at a time. Except for those times when I am completely unconscious (which I sometimes am), I do not let the fear hold me back from success, fulfillment and happiness.

If you are also committed to your success, fulfillment and happiness, then work on releasing your past attachments to fear. If you're still uncertain how to get "from here to there", Chapter Six will offer useful exercises to help in this process. Use the exercises outlined to begin the process of letting go of fear and moving on to your ultimate goal: happiness.

GUILT

Guilt can be a very painful feeling of self–reproach resulting from the belief that you have done something wrong or immoral. There can be any number of reasons you may feel guilty. You may believe that you should have taken precautions to avoid this pregnancy. Perhaps you were raised in an environment of strong religious convictions which directly oppose your single pregnancy. Maybe your family is displeased with you. Or, perhaps you considered, or even planned, to have an abortion and now feel guilty about allowing yourself to consider such a plan. You may even feel deserving of blame or punishment for allowing yourself to be in this predicament.

Your guilt needs healing and release. You will not feel freedom or personal joy as long as you have feelings of guilt over some facet of your life. Spending hours submerged in guilt will detract from your journey. So what can you do about the guilt?

Acknowledge that you feel it. Thank it for "sharing" and then do the work in this book to forgive yourself and get free from your attachment to guilt. Meditate for release. Pray for healing. Write a letter to your guilt; tell it you no longer need it. Write affirmations.

If you have harmed someone in any way and you feel guilty for your actions, this may be an indication that you need to go back and correct the problem. Perhaps an apology is warranted — or amends need to be made. Sometimes our guilt is telling us we need to take steps to redress a problem of our own making.

To some of you these approaches will be second nature. For others, they may seem contrite or even silly. But I suggest that if you are holding on to guilt, those feelings will only serve to hinder your growth and happiness.

CHAPTER SIX

YOUR MIND AND SPIRIT

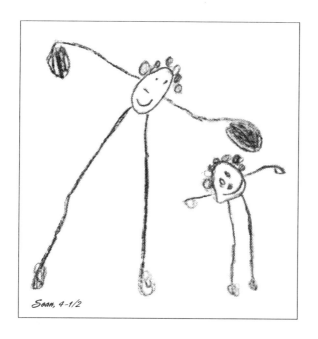

Sean, 4-1/2

WORKING ON A HEALTHY ATTITUDE: HOW YOUR BELIEFS AFFECT YOUR ATTITUDE

A healthy and good mental attitude does not always come naturally or without effort for any of us, especially when we are pregnant. We often have to work conscientiously at achieving it.

> *And life is what we make it,*
> *always has been, always will be.*
> Grandma Moses

How do my beliefs affect my attitude?

The ability to control your experiences – or at least your reaction to them – both during and after your pregnancy is rooted in your own mind and how you direct your thinking. Essentially, your beliefs are expectations or convictions that certain things are true or real. This being the case, you will find that the more positive energy you put into a particular way of seeing or believing in things, the more power you direct toward its manifestation.

Using your mind in concert with creative or positive thinking will produce positive results. The opposite is true as well. The more negative thinking (energy) you direct toward a particular situation, the more likely you are to see negative results. This may seem far–fetched, but it is true. Beliefs = experience. And beliefs ultimately affect our feelings — and even our moods.

For example, if you believe that your pregnancy will be difficult, you will consciously or unconsciously look for and manifest difficulty at every turn. Undoubtedly, you will discover exactly what you predetermined you would find; a difficult pregnancy. If however, you believe your pregnancy will be filled with joy and will progress smoothly, you are more apt to experience a joyful, smooth pregnancy.

Do my beliefs affect my physical health?

Yes. Your health and the quality of your pregnancy will be affected by the creative or positive thinking you direct toward it; or conversely, by the negative, self–defeating energy you direct toward it. This idea is now widely corroborated by psychosomatic medicine, with many well respected physicians acknowledging that the mind directly influences physical health and well–being.

Research indicates that the relationship between the unborn fetus and the parent (or parents) begins at conception, because your unborn baby shares your emotions at a psychological and hormonal level. Your stressful, negative thoughts and perceptions, whether they be about the general circumstances in your life, or specifically about your baby and/or your ability to care for him, can and do affect your health and that of your unborn child.

Further research indicates that negative thoughts and resulting stress contribute to increased autonomic nervous activity which in turn affects a part of your brain. This increase in autonomic nervous activity causes tension in the muscles and directly affects the flow of certain glands.

If you are experiencing stress and/or negative feelings, your pituitary gland will secrete a hormone (ACTH) which will cause your adrenal gland to release other hormones (cortisone and adrenaline–like substances). These hormones will cross the placental barrier and enter into the bloodstream of the baby, which in turn, can adversely affect your fetus. Likewise, the increased level of heart rate, respiratory rate, muscular tension, metabolic rate, and acid–base balance which are directly affected by the emotions (negative or positive) experienced by the mother, will also affect the unborn baby.

During pregnancy, it can be very difficult to "keep a stiff upper lip" and work at feeling good when you just don't feel you have the spirit in you to do so. Still, it is important to continually work consciously at maintaining a healthy attitude and to relieve as much of the stress and tension in your life as is possible for yours and your baby's good health and well–being.

Yea, that's easy for you to say, but I've got big problems!

It is perfectly natural for you to feel overwhelmed. You may feel sad or angry that your baby's father is not there to take care of you; or to cheer you on when days are tough. Maybe you feel vulnerable and uncertain about your future, and blame him for jumping ship. Perhaps you're worried about the financial burden of having this child. There are any number of reasons you may be feeling frightened, confused or depressed right now.

Within a normal range, (i.e., not constant or seriously depressed), these emotions are normal reactions to your situation. These feelings should not be construed as a weakness or sign that you are not handling this pregnancy as you "should".

Pregnancy is a tough time for any woman to go through — even if she's married or coupled and has the benefit of that extra support. Once you recognize that you are feeling a particular negative emotion, again, the question becomes "What can I do to turn this around?"

Eliminating the "power" struggle.

If, for example, your baby's father is giving you a hard time because (fill in the blank), though you cannot change his behavior, you *can* change your behavior. With awareness, you can choose how you respond to him, rather than reacting automatically.

This may be hard for you to swallow. Your instincts may be to fight back, to hurt him, or to keep fueling the problems between you. But, if you drop the ball in the middle of the game, the game stops. As much as you may want to "teach him a lesson," if you choose not to engage in unnecessary conflicts, you will be free to devote your attention and energies to your child and yourself.

Unfortunately, our relationships often trigger dysfunctional childhood patterns. And in some instances, counseling may be required to resolve them. In any case, as you learn to resolve these patterns, and eliminate conflicts, your thoughts and actions can then be used in a more loving and constructive ways.

This idea applies to money matters, career, family, friends, health, and any other situation you can name. You can learn to retrain your thoughts so that they work toward your good rather than undermining your efforts.

Sound crazy? Sound impossible? Perhaps. But this approach can work. You can use meditation, relaxation, visualization, affirmations, journaling, prayer, therapy, and any number of other techniques and resources to help you realize the power of your own abilities to create a positive life for yourself. However, you must first *want* to achieve these goals.

Willingness *and* effort is the key.

You must desire to be happy to such a degree that you are willing to do whatever it takes to fulfill your potential. The process of corrective action requires real effort and work on your part. If you don't take action, but expect things to change on their own, they probably won't. Learning to let go of negativity, and create a better and more loving experience, begins within *you*.

Take a look at the negative thoughts you choose to hold about any given situation in your life. Now look at what you can do about it. While you may not feel that a situation is good or fair, that does not mean that you can't adjust your thinking and take action to change yourself, change the situation, or both. Again, it is counterproductive for you to ask "Why me?" or to hold on to negative thoughts. This is the time for you to take action toward finding a resolution to the problems in your life.

Taking specific steps to transform your outlook and promote emotional well–being may seem comfortable and easy some of the time and overwhelming at other times. Whether you are positive and optimistic about your circumstance or you are full of fear and uncertainty, the results of your positive action will be enriching and rewarding whatever the outcome. We grow to greater heights when we stretch our boundaries.

Your attitude and feelings about your pregnancy may already be happy, healthy and optimistic. If that is the case, the suggestions herein can only serve to enhance an already positive experience. If, however, you are feeling lonely, isolated, afraid, stressed, (pick an adjective), try practicing some of the suggestions in this chapter. They *will* work!

DEEP BREATHING/MEDITATION

How can meditation help me?

During your pregnancy (and after), deep breathing and meditation are wonderful tools which can help you to relax and regroup. Meditation can also improve your sense of emotional well–being, and spiritual consciousness by redirecting your inner voices and thoughts toward peaceful, tranquil, positive and loving messages.

Meditation and meditative thought will also help to promote bonding between you and your unborn child. By using this technique, you can channel wonderfully positive and peaceful energy into your heart and mind.

Though there are many meditation techniques, the one I outline in this chapter involves pondering, reflecting, or studying a continuous thought. Meditation can be in the form of a written meditative thought or it can be oral, and works best when done on a continuous, daily basis.

How can I learn more about meditation?

To perfect the technique, meditation takes diligent practice to achieve deeper levels of relaxation and comfort. If you are not familiar with the practice of meditation, there are a variety of terrific books and tapes you can pick up at your local bookstore to help you better understand the purpose and practice of meditation. By reading and self–study, or through attending classes, you can practice and experiment with different techniques to find out which best suits you.

Additionally, I have produced meditation audio tapes which are specifically designed for you to listen to during your single pregnancy, and after, as a single mother. These tapes will help you with the meditation process (see last page of this book to order tapes). The first of these tapes, *Meditation and Your Unborn Child*, contains meditative thoughts for use during your pregnancy. The second tape, *Mother's Meditation*, is designed for use after your baby is born — though I lovingly refer to it as "When You are Pulling Your Hair Out".

Getting started.

For the process outlined in this section, set aside 15–20 minutes some time during the day to sit quietly with a meditative thought. Make sure the children, phones, television, and other potential interruptions will not disturb you during these sessions. This should be your own special quiet time.

It is best to sit up during these meditative sessions instead of lying down. Find a comfortable sitting position either in a chair or on a pillow or cushion on the floor. Unfold your legs and arms, and rest your hands on your lap with palms open. Gently close your eyes and allow your body to become relaxed. If it helps, play some peaceful instrumental music or nature sounds quietly in the background.

Focus on your breathing.

Begin your meditation with very relaxed breathing. Take a deep breath in and feel it fill your abdomen. Hold it for a moment to allow the breath to oxygenate your entire body. Then slowly let it out. As you inhale, imagine that the fresh breath is clearing out all the stress, fear, difficulties, and worries of your day. With each breath you take in, see these old energies evaporating.

As you exhale, release the residue of negativity out into the open air, freeing yourself from all the burdens you've been carrying in your heart and mind. Allow the exhaled breath to take away any anger or pent–up resentments you may be holding on to. In with the good air — out with the bad. Continue several times to breathe in — hold it — and breathe out, breathe in — hold it — and breathe out.

A Meditative thought.

Below is one suggested meditative thought which you can repeat to yourself in order to better calm and direct your thoughts.

Invite your mind and body to become still, quiet and tranquil. You can practice repeating this thought to yourself until you memorize it, or record it on tape using your own voice so you can sit and listen to it with your eyes closed. You may even want to create your own meditative thoughts. The point is to have a thought process which guides you to peace and tranquility, and which ultimately allows you to clear your mind of surface "chatter".

Repeat:

As I CLOSE MY EYES, I ALLOW MY BODY TO BECOME STILL, COMFORTABLE AND DEEPLY RELAXED. IN MY MIND'S EYE, I PAINT A PICTURE OF A BEAUTIFUL, QUIET AND RESTFUL PLACE WHERE I AM BATHED IN PEACE AND LOVE. I SEE CLEARLY AND VIVIDLY A FULL AND LUSH GARDEN OF BRIGHT, ILLUMINATING COLORS. THERE ARE GENTLE, FLOWING RIVERS OF LIQUID BLUE WATER SUCH AS I HAVE NEVER SEEN BEFORE. THE SOUNDS I HEAR ARE SWEET, AND SO LOVELY THAT I CANNOT HEAR THE SOUNDS OF ANYTHING OUTSIDE OF THIS HEAVENLY PLACE.

I NOW PLACE MYSELF IN THE GARDEN. I ALLOW MYSELF TO WALK IN THIS QUIET AND TRANQUIL PLACE WHICH I HAVE CREATED FOR MY GOOD AND PEACE. I SEE MYSELF VENTURING FURTHER AND FURTHER INTO MY GARDEN, AND AS I TRAVEL, I BECOME MORE AND MORE RELAXED.

I NOW SEE FORMING IN MY MIND'S EYE A GLOWING BALL OF BRILLIANT WHITE LIGHT. AS I FOCUS ON THE WHITE LIGHT, IT BECOMES LARGER, WARMER AND FULL OF MORE ENERGY THAN I HAVE EVER FELT OR EXPERIENCED BEFORE. THE WARMTH AND ENERGY OF THIS BRILLIANT WHITE LIGHT, WHICH FEELS SO GOOD AND COMFORTING, BEGINS TO SURROUND ME. IT FINALLY ENGULFS ME UNTIL I KNOW WITH CERTAINTY THAT I AM SAFE, WARM AND LOVED.

AS THIS WHITE LIGHT SURROUNDS ME, IT ALSO SURROUNDS MY BEAUTIFUL, PRECIOUS UNBORN BABY WHO IS FLOATING PEACEFULLY IN THE WARM AND GENTLE WATERS OF MY WOMB. THE WHITE LIGHT TOUCHES AND HOLDS SAFELY WITHIN ALL OF ITS BOUNTIFUL ENERGIES, MY UNBORN BABY. AND THIS LOVELY, PRECIOUS CHILD KNOWS AND FEELS THAT IT IS WANTED AND LOVED BY ME. TOGETHER, WE BASK IN THIS LIGHT WHILE GIVING AND RECEIVING LOVE TO ONE ANOTHER. IN THIS MOMENT WE ARE ONE, BECOMING CO–CREATORS OF HARMONY, JOY AND PEACE.

I CONTINUE TO HOLD THESE IMAGES IN MY MIND, AND ALLOW ANY OTHER UNINVITED THOUGHTS TO BE RELEASED IN FAVOR OF SILENCE AND STILLNESS.

When you have completed this meditative thought, keep your eyes closed and your body relaxed, while moving even more deeply into the peaceful atmosphere that you have created.

Release and relax.

Don't be discouraged if thoughts such as your grocery or "to do" list comes into your head as you attempt to meditate. It is natural for such uninvited thoughts to come into your mind. Do not dwell upon them or feel as if you are doing something wrong. Simply allow your mind to release these outside thoughts and redirect your attention to peace and stillness.

Again, it may be helpful to focus on your breathing. Having such a focus can help you stay centered and relaxed so that you are less easily distracted by mental chatter and can rapidly return to your own calm center. Sometimes counting breaths is helpful.

I usually remain quiet and still for approximately 15–20 minutes, but there is no correct or proper time limit. When you are ready to come back to your normal state, gently remind yourself that you are protected, loved and guided, and then slowly open your eyes to adjust to the here and now.

Meditation is about shifting our focus away from those intrusive, negative thoughts we often have (our problems, resentments, etc.) It's a good practice for daily life. It trains us to stay alert to where our mind is focusing so we can turn from negativity toward peace, love and stillness.

Mini–meditations.

If you are experiencing conflict in your day, perhaps at work, or with friends, family, etc., you can take a moment to re–center yourself utilizing the practice of meditation. Stop what you're doing, take some very deep cleansing breaths to circulate the oxygen in your body, and do a short, silent meditation — even if it's at your desk at work. A few minutes to quiet your thoughts can do wonders, and can help to bring you back to center.

RELAXATION AND VISUALIZATION TECHNIQUES

Almost all methods of natural childbirth use relaxation techniques to help the mother to be as mentally and physically comfortable as possible during labor. If you are stressed or tense throughout your pregnancy, you will likely experience a more uncomfortable pregnancy than if you are calm and relaxed. Likewise, if you have tensed muscles during your labor, you will likely have more discomfort throughout labor and delivery than is necessary.

How can relaxation and visualization benefit me?

Techniques for relaxation and visualization can help you achieve greater comfort both during your pregnancy and throughout labor, by relieving muscle tension, emotional tension, anxieties and fears. Muscle relaxation will also enhance your circulation and alter your body's physiological condition.

Relaxation and visualization techniques can also be used to relax your body and mind when you are feeling anxious, angry, upset, unhappy or worried. When you are tired and/or just before you go to sleep in the evening you can use the following process to induce a deeper and more relaxed sleep. This will be particularly helpful when you are having trouble sleeping in the latter months of pregnancy.

Relaxation can also benefit you if you are feeling sick or physically uncomfortable. But the technique does require practice on your part to help you enjoy deeper levels of relief from these discomforts.

A better perspective.

Did you know that when you are relaxed you actually perceive things differently than when you are tense and rigid? By altering your stress and tension level to a more relaxed state, you brighten your outlook and benefit yourself and your baby – physically and emotionally.

Getting started.

To get started, lie in a comfortable position with your legs uncrossed, and your arms resting at your sides. Take in a few deep breaths through your nose, breathing the air into your diaphragm. Hold the breath for a moment and let the oxygen flow through your body.

Slowly and audibly release the breath through your mouth. Allow your abdomen to rise on the inhalation, and fall on the exhalation. Allow your limbs to remain loose and limp. Repeat this breathing process several times until you start to feel comfortable and relaxed.

For the next step, it might be a good idea to have someone read the following instructions to you at first (or audio tape them), until you are able to repeat these thoughts and directions to yourself by memory.

A mantra for relaxation:

Beginning with your feet, say to yourself: "My feet are relaxed. They are feeling more and more relaxed." Relax for a few moments. In your mind, see your feet as being relaxed. Experience how your feet feel in this relaxed state. Move now to your ankles, and repeat to yourself: "My ankles are relaxed. They are feeling more and more relaxed." Relax for a few moments. As you do so, see a picture in your mind of your ankles becoming more and more relaxed. Again, experience the sensation of your ankles in their relaxed state.

Move now to your calves, and repeat to yourself "My calves are relaxed. They are feeling more and more relaxed." Relax for a few moments. Visualize and experience your calves becoming more and more relaxed. Move now to your knees, and repeat "My knees are relaxed. They are feeling more and more relaxed." Relax for a few moments and visualize and experience your knees as being relaxed.

Now continue in the same process, moving to your upper thighs. When you relax your thighs, feel the sensations that relaxing causes in your muscles and visualize the process in your mind. In the same fashion, move to your pelvis. Relax, and visualize. Move to your abdomen and think of the baby floating in your uterus and relax. Imagine now, the baby, comfortable, healthy, and protected in the safety of your uterus.

Move now to your chest. Relax, and visualize. Move to your

back. Relax the muscles and tension in your back. Relax, and visualize. Move to your shoulders. Relax, and visualize. Move to your upper arms. Relax, and visualize. Move to your elbows. Relax. Move to your forearms. Relax. Move to your fingers, feel each finger on each hand relaxing. See each finger becoming more and more relaxed as you direct them to do so. Relax your neck. Relax your jaw. Allow your jaw to drop. Relax. Relax your tongue. Relax your cheeks. Relax your eyes. Relax your forehead. Relax the top of your head. Visualize each of these steps as your body becomes heavy, limp, and deeply relaxed.

Moving to a deeper state of relaxation.

You should now rest and allow yourself to feel the sensation of your entire body in its relaxed state. To move into a deeper state of relaxation, begin counting backwards from ten:

"Ten, I am feeling more relaxed." Take in a deep cleansing breath. As you exhale, continue: "Nine, I am feeling more relaxed." Take in another deep cleansing breath and on the exhale, continue "Eight, I am feeling more relaxed." Continue downward to zero.

You are now in a deeper and more relaxed state of being. Your body and mind feel peaceful. Your baby is also relaxed in this state. You may stay in this state for as long as you feel comfortable doing so.

When you are ready to return to your normal state of consciousness, slowly put your hands over your eyes. As you begin to open your eyes (very slowly now), you simultaneously open the space between your fingers to allow your eyes to adjust to the light. Then slowly stretch your arms, your fingers, your legs, toes and so on.

Improving technique through practice.

The more you practice any relaxation and visualization techniques the easier it will be to achieve deeper levels of calm and to experience subtle feelings within your body. If you do not feel that anything is happening the first few times you try this exercise, or if you feel silly or awkward doing it, do not let that discourage you. Something very real is happening to you that can even be measured scientifically.

RECEPTIVE VISUALIZATION

What is Receptive Visualization?

Receptive Visualization is a process where you allow, or invite, your mind to form "mental pictures" of its own thoughts and images. Before doing this exercise, however, you should familiarize yourself with the relaxation exercise described on page 86.

For maximum benefits, it's a good idea to go through the process of relaxing your body to its deepest state before doing Receptive Visualization. Later, as you become more accomplished at relaxing your body, you will find that abdominal breathing alone brings you to a sufficiently relaxed state in preparation of this exercise.

How can Receptive Visualization help me?

It is important for you to get in touch with your feelings about your pregnancy and becoming a (single) parent. Allowing your mind to be open and receptive to its own thoughts and images can help you to get in touch with your feelings about your pregnancy, as well as other things. It can also help you to find answers to the many questions you may have about your pregnancy and parenting experiences.

Getting started.

Find a comfortable place where you can relax and not be disturbed. This technique can be done while sitting or lying down, whichever is most comfortable for you. Close your eyes and begin by slowly breathing in and out — allowing your abdomen to rise and fall. After several deep cleansing breaths you will begin to feel relaxed.

You are now ready to open your mind to mental pictures relating to your feelings about your pregnancy; or perhaps your ideas about being a single–parent, etc. Imagine that your mind is a movie screen, able to project "scenes" which relate to your hopes, fears, and ideas about your pregnancy and/or labor, etc.

You may want to begin by visualizing your healthy baby in your womb. Take time to explore each facet of her beauty. See her eyes, nose, mouth, ears, fingers, toes, and tiny little body, etc. You can look at this image and elaborate upon it for as long as you like.

Another visualization process might include the kind of delivery you envision. Allow yourself to explore this image in as much detail as you can. The ideas you will have about pregnancy and parenting are endless. Choose appropriate "scenes" which depict your ideas or images about your life with your new baby, or the life you want with your child.

There are no "correct" ideas to have about your pregnancy or parenting, and no appropriate or inappropriate responses to those ideas. Our goal here, once again, is to have the most relaxed and enjoyable experience possible while gaining insight into our own feelings.

Some images may make you feel elated or happy; some may make you feel uncomfortable or sad. Try not to dwell upon these images, but simply to make a note of your experience or feelings about them. As you continue the practice of visualization, your ideas and feelings will flow more easily and become more clear to you.

When you open yourself up to this process, any number of feelings — and even old memories — may come up for you. Some may surprise you. "Where did that come from?" If troubling memories, worries or feelings come up, don't be discouraged. In fact, look upon them as opportunities to grow and to heal. If you can't seem to work through them on your own, it may be helpful to talk to a professional to help you resolve the conflict.

Another way to help absorb your strengths, let go of, or improve upon weaknesses and heal conflicts, is to do written and verbal affirmations (as outlined below).

AFFIRMATIONS

What is an affirmation?

An affirmation is a positive declaration. It can be a word, expression or statement intended to create, confirm or uphold positive ideas about yourself to yourself. Its intention here is to remind you to accept and believe in your own inherent goodness and capabilities.

We all need to be reminded that we are wonderful, terrific, valuable, vibrant women, *especially* when our hormones are raging and we are experiencing the everyday changes that pregnancies bring on. And, when you already have children under foot, you need to remind yourself that in addition to being "Mommy", you are a dynamic, sexy, beautiful woman.

You may want to affirm your value as an employee, boss, or businesswoman. You may want to affirm your worthiness of attracting a perfect mate, or finding happiness. Since presently at least, there's not a "him" there to encourage you and tell you all the wonderful things about you, you've got to remind yourself — and remind yourself often — how wonderful you really are.

Getting started.

It's a great idea to write out an affirmation, or two, or three, or four, or more, and tape them all over the house. Go crazy with it. Put one on the bathroom mirror; on the front door; on the refrigerator; on the steering wheel of your car, and anyplace else where you'll see it often. Here are a few suggestions for love notes to yourself:

"I am a beautiful, vibrant woman"
"Together, my baby and I are healthy,
happy and full of love"
"I can do anything I set my mind to"
"I am a wonderful, loving mother"
"Abundance is mine"

These are wonderful ways to remind yourself that you are a special and very powerful woman. It is so important to your outlook and attitude to know, to believe, and to feel that you are special. Choose affirmations for yourself that best fit your circumstances, needs or goals.

Another positive, affirmative action you can take is to write repetitive affirmations. If you are feeling unattractive in your pregnant state, write an affirmation about how beautiful you are! Maybe you are afraid of the responsibilities of being a single–parent. Write an affirmation about the upside or possibilities of your decision. The topics are endless.

Choose an affirmation that fits your needs, wants, or desires, and write it down 100 times. In the far right–hand column of the paper after each entry, write the first thought or belief about your written affirmation that comes to your mind.

Don't think too much about what comes up, or what thought to write. Simply allow your natural reactions to flow and your inner voice to speak. There are no right or wrong responses. An example of this might be:

Together my baby and I will flourish	*I believe*
Together my baby and I will flourish	*I'm afraid*
Together my baby and I will flourish	*We can*
Together my baby and I will flourish	*I feel silly*
Together my baby and I will flourish	*I'm alone*
Together my baby and I will flourish	*I'm never really alone*
Together my baby and I will flourish	*I can do this!*

Assessing your responses.

When you have completed your writing, take a look at the right hand column entries. What kind of pattern has developed? Are your reactive thoughts more positive? More negative? A combination of both? You may not have been consciously aware of many of your deeper feelings.

As you review your responses, you can better see what issues you need to address – where to give yourself credit – and where to do some inner work. As you address your fears and negativity with insight, compassion and action, you will be able to replace painful feelings and destructive beliefs with positive ones quite naturally.

You owe it to yourself and to your baby to try to forgive whatever real or perceived injustices you feel have been perpetrated against you by people in your life, including yourself. You aren't excusing the behavior. You may even need to take action (legal or otherwise). But holding on to negative emotions is unhealthy for you and your baby. So write an affirmation on acceptance and forgiveness.

WRITING

Begin to keep a daily journal or diary of your thoughts, feelings, and experiences about your pregnancy, the baby growing inside of you, and life in general. Writing is a great way to release negative energy, to document wonderful experiences, to get clear on your feelings, and to give yourself credit for your victories.

Your writing does not have to be perfect, literary, or grammatically correct. Just get it out. Have a good time with it; or even a good cry. The point is to release feelings and ideas so they do not stay bottled up inside of you.

Write when you are happy and feeling great, and write when you are sad or angry. Either way, writing is a tool you can utilize to release and express your truest feelings in a positive and constructive way.

A special gift - *Love letters to a child.*

Among the most precious gifts I have ever given to myself (and someday I will give these gifts to each of my sons), are baby books that I have been writing to them since I was pregnant with each of them. For my eldest son, Taylor, I bought one of those hard–bound books with crisp, empty white pages in it (it had a white canvas cover and so I personalized it by painting funny little animals on it with acrylic paints). In this book, I write down poems, feelings, experiences; the funny things he does or says; and my feelings on life, love and the pursuit of happiness. I even write to him when I am sad.

I figure that when Taylor grows up and I am able to give this book to him, he will be able to know me better than just who he perceives me to be, because my writing in the journal is unedited, spontaneous and so very intimate. Perhaps some of the things I write to him in this journal will be told to him time and time again in his life. But then again, some of the little things might slip by and I may never say them. By writing these very special thoughts to him, I'm letting him know me and my heart.

I plan to wait until he is at least 16 or 17 to give him the book – –or maybe when he's 21. The appropriate time will undoubtedly announce itself to me. I do not write every day in this book. Sometimes once a month, sometimes less and sometimes more. When I feel the urge, I just write.

I also started a book for Jace, my second son, before he was born. Because he is so young, not much has been written. But the remaining empty pages are waiting to be filled with all of the special things I have to say to this brilliant, unique, and wonderful child.

Consider writing your own journal or baby book for your child. This gift to your child will be unlike any other, because it will be a one–of–a–kind, intimate view of his mother as well as a chronicle of his own development. He will undoubtedly appreciate this special effort when he's old enough to understand the love and attention that went into creating it.

Writing a "therapeutic" letter.

Another idea which I found to be therapeutic is to write a letter to anyone with whom you may have some unresolved issues. It could be a letter to the baby's father, to a friend or family member, or even your boss. This letter is not necessarily intended to be delivered or mailed. In fact, if it is an angry letter, I suggest that you keep it to yourself. The point of this exercise is not to lash out at others who may have hurt you, but to release your honest feelings of hurt and anger in order to let go of them and find love and healing for yourself.

Finding love and healing is so very important for you, your unborn child, and to your growing children. In fact, some consider these qualities to be the most important things we seek to find in our lifetimes.

Because our energies and attitudes (loving or otherwise) are projected to, and experienced by, our kids — even before they are born — it is all the more important that we possess these qualities. Our angry, resentful, or hurt feelings will find expression one way or another. To encourage growth, and to protect our children, we need to find positive outlets where we can vent these feelings constructively.

If you don't learn to release your negative feelings, it is highly unlikely that you will find any great measure of peace in your life. Instead, these feelings will simmer within you and sabotage your chances for happiness and fulfillment.

If you're feeling angry or upset, write about it! It's perfectly fine to write out angry or resentful thoughts in a letter or journal. It's far wiser to choose to release the anger than to keep it pent up, festering in your heart and mind.

No matter what our circumstances, life will bring us challenges and upsets — and these feelings need to find healthy expression. The ultimate goal is to release the negative feelings we carry with us so that they don't contaminate our lives and the lives of our children.

Writing as an on–going form of release.

Utilizing the tool of writing will not only help you when you are pregnant, but will help you throughout your life. It is an invaluable form of self–help therapy and self–expression. And in looking back on what you have written, you will have the means to chart your progress and accomplishments.

PRAYER

Prayer and the subject of God and Spirituality is a very personal matter. But I would feel remiss in not mentioning what, in my experience, has been a very powerful tool of healing and growth. You may or may not be religious or spiritual.

I'm not a religious fanatic; and I am certainly not trying to convert anyone here. We each must find our own faith and way to exercise it. However, I do want to share that prayer has been a very powerful tool in my life's journey; especially where my mothering is concerned. When used on a daily basis, it has helped me to remember why I am here and what is important in my life. Prayer helps me when I am feeling afraid and lonely because it enables me to sense the larger presence that is always with me. Prayer is also important to me when times are good, reminding me to keep centered.

My prayers remind me that there is a plan in all of this (babies, life, love, tragedies, etc.) and that life has more meaning to it than sometimes appears on the surface of things. Prayer also keeps me humble when my head gets to too big, or when I forget what is most important. In fact, the power of prayer reminds me of what I sometimes forget: that I am loved, I am worthy, I am wonderful.

Spirituality: A medical miracle?

Some scientists are also beginning to take a serious look at just what benefits patients may derive from spirituality and prayer. Much to their surprise, they are finding a good deal of relevant data buried in medical literature that offers evidence that a strong spiritual life is good for one's health.

According to Dr. Herbert Benson, president of Mind/Body Medical Institute of Boston's Deaconess Hospital and Harvard Medical School, prayer affects the "stress hormones", leading to lower blood pressure, more relaxed heart rate and respiration among other benefits. Other studies have shown that men and women who attend church regularly have been found to have less heart disease, lower rates of depression and generally better health than those who do not attend.

It sometimes takes faith to find your faith.

If you have trouble with the concept of God but you can see that there is something in the universe that is greater than us — a Higher Power — try praying to that power. Pray not only when your back is up against the wall, but do so simply to give thanks for all of your blessings. Counting blessings can be an excellent antidote to the blues.

The Serenity Prayer is a non–denominational prayer that has a very simple and humble request of God, Higher Power, or the creative energies of the universe:

*G*RANT ME THE SERENITY
TO ACCEPT THE THINGS I CANNOT CHANGE,
COURAGE TO CHANGE THE THINGS I CAN,
AND THE WISDOM TO KNOW THE DIFFERENCE

When I hear, and I *really* attempt to understand the words of this simple prayer, I realize that its message covers the basic dilemmas I have in my life. I sometimes overlook what I can do something about, and I'm not always very wise about what I can or cannot change.

Do you see yourself in there somewhere? This prayer asks for something so basic. Simply, that we become consciously aware of what we can and cannot control, and find acceptance about it. I utilize this prayer, when things seem to become too complicated for me. It reminds me to turn my problems over to the Powers that Be in the universe.

THERAPY/COUNSELING

If you are feeling anxiety, depression or any other degree of emotional discomfort which feels too difficult to handle on your own, by all means, go see a therapist or psychologist. A trained professional can help you to better understand and deal with your problems.

I'm not "sick" and I don't need a therapist!

Many people are reluctant to seek help because they see it as a sign of weakness. Others think only "crazy" or "sick" people see mental health professionals. These perceptions couldn't be further from the truth. People who seek help from counselors have a fundamental strength. They value themselves enough to take care of their lives. They also possess the desire and will to overcome their challenges.

Seeking help from a professional does not mean you are "weak", "crazy", or "sick". You are a terrific person with a lot going on right now. You may simply need some intervention to help you deal more effectively with your situation.

What to look for in a counselor or therapist.

When choosing a counselor or therapist, it is important that you are comfortable with, and feel secure about this person. Do they appear to be a sympathetic listener? What is their demeanor? Do you prefer a man or woman? Trust your feelings and intuitions. If your instincts tell you the person is not right for you, look into finding a more suitable counselor or therapist.

Ask the professional about their credentials and area(s) of specialty. How long have they been practicing in their field? Find out if their schedule is available to meet your own. Ask about their cancellation policy if you must miss an appointment due to an emergency or illness.

Finding referrals.

For referrals, ask your friends or doctor whom they recommend. You can also request a referral to a therapist in your area from the National Mental Health Association,(703) 684–7722.

Try contacting your local free clinic. Many of them offer mental health services free or for a nominal charge. Your local crisis pregnancy center can also refer you to a counselor (and help you with other services too).

Look in your yellow pages under the heading "Social Services Organizations", or "Social Workers". Pro–life organizations may also be able to refer you to counselors in your area. Your church or synagogue can likely provide resources or referrals to you as well. For additional referrals, look in the Resource Section at the end of this book.

I found assistance during my second pregnancy under the listing "abortion alternatives" in the yellow pages. The pregnancy crisis center I contacted offered a variety of services for pregnant women. They were very helpful and supportive, and provided me with terrific referrals. Leave no stone unturned. If you need help, be creative. Seek it wherever you can find it.

If your insurance doesn't cover therapy sessions, ask a potential therapist if they work on a sliding scale. Many therapists will adjust their fee according to your ability to pay. So, ask what kind of arrangements you can make with them.

MUSIC AND BUBBLE BATH "THERAPY"

As a working woman who is always on the go, I had to create relaxation time for myself. I found that one of the most beneficial ways for me to relax was when I was in the tub. This meant I was not talking on the phone, doing chores, working, painting, or any of the numerous other things that constantly keep me busy and on the go.

If you, too, are busy and on the go in your own daily life, try to slow down long enough to enjoy "bubble bath therapy". Bubble baths — or aromatic herbs — are terrific! But there are some rules:

Rule number one: When you are pregnant, make sure the water is not too hot, as it is very unhealthy for your fetus, especially during the first few months.

Rule number two: If you turn on the stereo, do not listen to love songs or music that makes you sad if you are feeling vulnerable! It isn't emotionally healthy for you. Turn your radio to a more upbeat station, perhaps rock n' roll, jazz, classical or new age. When you do hear a song that makes you feel unhappy, if you can't turn it off, work to retrain your mind about its meaning. For instance, learn to sing the love song to your baby. Sing along as if each word was written especially for your child or beautiful new baby. I used to sing *I'll Always Love You,* by Taylor Dane to my first son while he was in my tummy. That's how he came to be called Taylor.

Rule number three: Relax. Pamper yourself. Close your eyes and soak for awhile. Let Calgon take you away. Add some bath salts for a lengthy luxury bath, and take that time in the tub to relax, perhaps indulging in some meditation or visualization techniques.

Rule number four: Enjoy yourself!

Besides good and adequate hygiene being absolutely essential during your pregnancy, this relaxation time is beneficial for both you and your unborn baby. Mornings are an especially good time for baths, as they help to get your day off to a very soothing start. But a good soak at the end of the evening can take the edge off a stressful day.

Bathing with your baby.

When Taylor was a newborn he hated his little blue plastic bath tub and screamed loudly every time I put him in it. But he loved — *I mean really loved* — taking a bath with me. So there was no contest. He took baths with me for the first few years.

Bathing together was another way for us to bond and to spend special time together on my restrictive time budget. We had some wonderful times together playing and singing in the tub. You may be more conventional than I am, or this approach may not be appropriate for you, but you won't know unless you try it.

Giving up our bathtime together was harder for me than giving up breast–feeding. I decided in advance that I would stop bathing with Taylor when he was at an age where it became embarrassing for him; when he started to make a big deal out of our gender differences; or when he was clearly too old to continue.

Ultimately, Taylor never became embarrassed about his or my anatomy, and he never made a big deal over our gender differences – probably because I didn't either. I discussed our differences freely, and answered his questions honestly and openly without much ado. That probably contributed to his nonchalance on the subject. He became too old to bathe with me long before he cared about our anatomical differences. We stopped bathing together when Taylor was nearly four.

I am continuing the tradition with my little one, Jace. Each morning before I go off to work, we jump in the tub for a 15 minute bath together. It has now become one of our special bonding times together and, like Taylor, he loves it!

Note: For many, the subject of bathing with a child may be controversial because of the issues we face in our society concerning sexual abuse. This section is written from the perspective that bathing with your infant or toddler is a bonding process of love and sharing. It assumes that the reader is a "healthy" individual, who understands appropriate boundaries and behaviors toward her children.

STRESS

Harmful effects of stress:

Stress is defined in Webster's New World Dictionary as "a strain or straining force...exerted upon a body, that tends to strain or deform its shape..." Sounds lovely doesn't it? But that's just what stress is doing to us.

Research also indicates that prolonged, high levels of stress in pregnant mothers, produce higher numbers of babies with low birth weights. Furthermore, women who experience severe emotional distress or depression during their pregnancies commonly have babies who are colicky, hyperactive, restless, and irritable.

We have been hearing for sometime about how stress causes illness and injury to our bodies, and emotional distress to our minds. But what can we do to eliminate stress? First of all, we need to identify the stress that exists in our lives. We then need to determine what we can do to help eliminate as much of it as is possible. The trick sometimes is to figure out the source of the stresses in our lives.

The obvious – and not–so–obvious stresses of our lives.

Stress can emanate from obvious and not such obvious places. It can come from our jobs, financial situations, families, children, relationships (friends and lovers), the death of a loved one, among many other situations. These sources are easily identified as stressful situations. But stress can also be caused by everyday situations or circumstances that we may not even realize are contributing to our overall tenseness. For example, moving to a new home or new job, birthdays, holidays, world politics, city congestion, traffic — and yes, single–parenting — to name just a few. Take a look at your life and see where stress may exist.

Letting go of stress.

Of course nobody can live stress–free. Stress is a part of life and living. However, we can choose to eliminate unnecessary stresses in our lives. It's not always easy, but it's certainly possible. Perhaps a bad relationship is keeping you in the revolving door. Maybe it's time to let it go. If family is a problem for you, see less of them. If your job is too stressful, look into other possibilities.

Holding on to stress.

At the same time, look closely at the stressors you have and see if you have an interest in keeping the drama in your life. For many of us, although we claim to desire happiness, we are subconsciously attracted to high drama; and drama causes stress.

You might be saying "Keri is nuts. I don't like, or attract drama and stress in my life!" Well, that may or may not be true. But it is worth looking into. What situations do you continue to recreate in your life? What are the possible pay–offs for keeping certain uncomfortable relationships or situations in your life? What is your part in creating the stresses around you? Looking at the answers to these questions can enlighten us and encourage constructive change.

Into action.

Obviously these are some simple suggestions to very complex problems. And taking action to change our circumstances can seem difficult or nearly impossible at times. But once we make a decision to change our circumstances, things can be different if we really want them to be different. But only if we take action.

I have found that when I'm so overwhelmed by circumstances which I no longer choose to accept in my life, that I am most willing (and ready) to take action to change those circumstances. It has also been helpful for me to be willing to see my part in allowing certain things to be created in my life.

It is unfortunate that many of us need to have our backs up against the wall in order to get seriously motivated to make alterations in our lives. Pain is indeed a great motivator.

Steps toward change.

We do not need to make drastic changes all at once (this too can and will cause more stress). But we can make changes and alterations in slow measures.

Make a list of the things in your life that cause you anxiety and/ or stress. Then look for creative ways to eliminate the unnecessary stresses of your every day life.

Start with the less challenging situations which can be more easily remedied: Perhaps you're too tired to clean your house and do your laundry and you've been putting it off for days (or even weeks). How about enlisting a friend to come over and help you? In traffic, learn deep breathing techniques, or listen to motivational tapes or music. Learn to better manage your time and prioritize your daily affairs. Take a stress–reduction course. Practice yoga. Clear up conflicts with friends and family.

As you rid yourself of the lesser stresses, begin to work your way up to the bigger issues. But don't take on too much at one time. Use the techniques in this book, such as meditation, affirmations, exercise, positive imaging, etc. to help you learn to let go of stress. In some instances, counseling may be beneficial to help you deal with certain issues you can't handle on your own.

SUPPORT GROUPS

I feel as if I'm all alone in my predicament. Where can I turn for help?

There will very likely be times when you feel that you are all alone. You may feel that nobody could possibly understand what you are going through. Fortunately, there are many resources available to you. In addition to your friends and family, there are women's groups, single–parent groups, counseling services, licensed therapists, physicians, practitioners, and clergy, among others to help you get through the next nine months.

Where two or more are gathered...

There is definitely power in numbers! One of the greatest inspirations throughout both of my pregnancies — and often in my parenting experience — has been the support of other women (and sometimes even single fathers) who were in the same, or similar situation as I.

Although in many ways mothering came quite naturally and instinctively to me, I still found at times that I felt afraid, awkward and unsure of myself. The single mothers who embraced and helped me through those early years really helped me to overcome my fears and to become a better parent.

Finding a support group is one way to help you see that you are not alone in your predicament. A support group can remind you that there are others just like you who, against many odds, are doing a wonderful job of raising their children on their own. Other single–parents can also offer you a variety of information and tips about their own experiences which may help you in your situation.

Support groups are a great forum to discuss your fears, concerns and problems, as well as a place to share the bright and positive sides of your pregnancies and parenting experiences. Here are some organizations which may be helpful to you:

NATIONAL ORGANIZATION OF SINGLE MOTHERS, INC.(NOSM)

This is a non–profit organization committed to helping single–parents meet the challenges of daily life with wisdom, dignity, courage and humor. The group was founded by Andrea Engber, who is also a single mother. NOSM seeks to empower families and to unite them in a network of mutual support and action through its publication *SingleMOTHER*, by establishing nationwide support groups.

A one year membership in NOSM is $15.00 (or $12.80) for low–income women). A subscription to *SingleMOTHER* is included with membership. You can contact NOSM by writing to: P.O. Box 68, Midland, North Carolina 28107–0068. Information on local chapters is available by calling (704) 888–KIDS.

PARENTS PLACE: THE PARENTING RESOURCE CENTER ON THE WEB

Parents Place is a home business on the Web. It operates under the belief that parents are the best resource for other parents. They offer articles on pregnancy, breast–feeding, baby, adolescence, parenting twins, step–parenting, single–parenting, children's health and education, family activities, and more. They also offer opportunities for parenting dialog (live chat or public E–mail) and for shopping. They can be located on the Web at: http://www.parentsplace.com/.

SINGLE MOTHERS BY CHOICE (SMC)

Founded by Dr. Jane Mattes, a psychotherapist and single mother, SMC is a nonprofit organization that provides information and support to single mothers as well as to those contemplating or trying to achieve single motherhood.

Members of SMC tend to be financially secure career women, who chose to become single mothers. The decision may have been made as a result of an accidental pregnancy, intentional conception or adoption.

A national membership fee is $45.00 for the first year, and includes a membership directory for your area and the name of a local contact person. It also includes an information package containing resources for adoption and donor insemination, as well as a one–year subscription to the SMC quarterly newsletter. The newsletter can be ordered separately for $20.00. Membership renewal fees are $30.00 per year.

To find out more about SMC, write to Single Mothers by Choice, P.O. Box 1642, Gracie Square Station, New York, New York 10028, or call (212) 988–0993. You can also E–mail SMC at: mattes@pipline.com.

THE NURTURING NETWORK

The Nurturing Network was founded by Mary Cunningham Agee, a Harvard Business School graduate and former venture capitalist. The organization is dedicated to helping all women, but particularly those who are college educated or career oriented to deal with unplanned pregnancies.

Services include counseling, housing with member families, financial assistance, medical referrals, client–employer mediation, mentor programs, adoption counseling and services, college transfers, parenting classes and child care referrals.

For more information, write to The Nurturing Network, 200 Clocktower Place, Suite 200A, P.O. Box 223099, Carmel, California 93922, or call (800) TNN– 4MOM.

PARENTS WITHOUT PARTNERS INTERNATIONAL, INC. (PWP)

Parents Without Partners is an international organization that promotes activities for single–parents (both men and women) and their kids. PWP addresses social, educational, and advocacy issues of single–parents. Although most members already have children, single pregnant women have joined PWP before their babies were born.

PWP activities include such things as trips to baseball games, bowling, picnics, parties, etc. Many of the groups (chapters) also hold weekly discussions for parents on varying topics which are hosted in members' homes. Some activities are "adult only", while other events include the kids.

The annual membership fee varies depending on the local chapter, but is in the range of 35.00 per year. Activities generally cost a few bucks or so to attend. Membership also includes a subscription to *Single Parent* magazine. To find out more about PWP, write to Parents Without Partners, 401 North Michigan Avenue, Chicago, Illinois 60611, or call (312) 644–6610.

THE NATIONAL BLACK WOMEN'S HEALTH PROJECT (NBWHP)

The National Black Women's Health Project was founded by Byllye Avery as a pilot program of the National Women's Health Network. NBWHP has local chapters in 31 states, with over 100 support groups across the country. NBWHP works to empower African American women who have grown "sick and tired of being sick and tired". Their aim is to create change by first changing their own lives, and then carry the message to other women.

Services include prenatal care, single mother self–help groups, job training, housing referrals, tutorial programs, and help in dealing with government aid programs. The organization also offers referrals to other sources of help and information. For referrals call NBWHP's help–line at (800) ASK–BWHP.

Membership in NBWHP is a $10, $25, $50, or $100 voluntary contribution, and is tax–deductible. For more details about NBWHP, write to: The National Black Women's Health Project, 1237 R.D. Abernathy Boulevard, SW, Atlanta, Georgia 30310, or call (404) 758–9590.

CARENET

CareNet is an organization of Christian women's centers dedicated to helping pregnant women in crisis who have decided to give birth to their babies. Though the group is Christian in approach, it helps all women without regard to their personal faith. Services include parenting classes, job training, financial advice, free maternity clothes and baby furniture, plus other referrals. For more information for assistance in your area, call (703) 478–5661.

PARENTS ANONYMOUS

This organization is the only national mutual support and parent self–help program effectively preventing child abuse and neglect. Services are provided free of charge to strengthen families through parent–led, professionally–facilitated groups for parents, and specialized programs for children. On any given week, over 15,000 parents come together in a Parents Anonymous group to resolve their problems and learn new ways to nurture their children and themselves. For more information about a Parents Anonymous group in your area, call (909) 621–6184.

SOLO – A Guide for the Single Parent – Newsletter

Solo is a bi–monthly newsletter, founded by single mother Marilyn Facey. *Solo* offers support, information, and discussions concerning a variety of important issues related to single–parenting. Subscriptions cost $18.00 per year. This resource is particularly helpful for women who live in remote areas that do not have a lot to offer in the way of support groups. To order, call (800) 477–5877.

YWCA

The Young Women's Christian Association (YWCA), while rooted in Christian philosophies, is open to women of all faiths. The YWCA offers prenatal exercise classes, child care, mommy and baby classes, support groups, career counseling, help for victims of abuse, plus many opportunities to socialize with other mothers. However, you will need to check with your local YMCA to see if they have the particular class you want, as each Y offers its own curriculum to women in the community. Check your white pages for the number of the YMCA closest to you, or call (212) 614–2700 to request a World-wide Directory.

Where can I find other resources?

For other organizations which may be of interest to you, look in your local papers, parenting magazines, neighborhood throw–always. Also check your local churches and hospitals for support groups.

You can also look in the yellow pages under the heading "So-cial Service Organizations", or in the "Subject Index". A variety of different organizations exist under these headings which may be very helpful to you. Sometimes the organization name or heading is vague, so if it sounds like they might have something to offer you, give them a call and ask them what their organization does.

Starting your own support group.

If you can't find a support group in your community, start one yourself! Forming a group will take a strong commitment on your part. But you will undoubtedly find that there are other single moth-ers in your area who will be thrilled to join with you.

Several years ago, I belonged to a support group of about eight single mothers. We met once a week to share our experiences and to encourage one another. We started out each group session with every woman taking a turn, having three minutes of uninterrupted time to talk about whatever was "up" for her during her week. Nobody was allowed to interrupt and there was no cross–talking during those three minutes.

Finally, after everybody was done, the group opened up to "free–talk" where we shared back and forth about whatever came up. The topics seemed to naturally present themselves, and we were never at a loss for words. At the close of the meeting, we discussed old and new business.

As a group, we held potluck dinners about once a month, went on outings with our kids, had garage sales, and had a barter system for trading goods and services. In this barter system, we used coins to trade one another for services such as massage, bookkeeping, painting, babysitting, etc.

The system worked well, as we all had something to contribute to one another. Eventually, I moved on from the group, but I have maintained friendships with several of the women from the group.

You can start a group of your own by placing an ad in local papers, community centers, day–care centers, etc. Or contact the Family Resource Coalition, 200 South Michigan Avenue, Suite 1520, Chicago, Illinois 60604, (312) 341–0900. They can provide you with a free copy of *"How to Start a Support Group,"* and literature on how to find family support programs in your area.

CHAPTER SEVEN

PREPARING FOR BABY

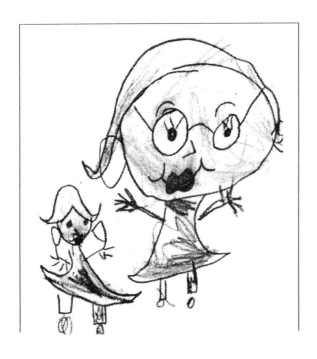

BONDING WITH YOUR UNBORN CHILD

The process of communicating and bonding with your baby actually begins long before she is born. Because your baby's initial primary attitudes are shaped by the messages she receives from you before she is born, your own attitude and feelings toward her are important. They will significantly contribute to, or detract from, the bonding process you share with your child. Your attitude — positive or negative — will also be the foundation upon which you establish the early relationship between you.

This feels like a dream!

At first, your pregnancy may seem more like a dream than reality. You may feel particularly close to your unborn child, or she may be as remote to you as a relative you've never met. Both reactions are normal.

As your body changes and your stomach grows to accommodate the growing fetus within you, so too will your awareness that this is for real. Your emotional attachment to this child has begun — there really is a baby there!

Communication with your unborn child.

Talking and singing to your unborn child will help you to relate to her as a real person. As a result of talking and singing during pregnancy, your baby will learn to recognize the sound of your voice. She will know you instantly after her birth. And she will be soothed by the comforting sound of hearing you speak or sing. Rubbing and holding your tummy, and thinking "pink fuzzy" thoughts are also expressions of the process of bonding.

Giving your baby a "pet" name while you are still pregnant may also enhance the quality of your relationship to your baby. By referring to your unborn child with a pet name (such as "Thumper", "Peanut", etc.), she is no longer simply an "it". She becomes more real –

– more of a person.

Many people assume that a baby is not really there until it is born. This is not true at all! During the stages of your baby's development, researchers have found that babies function, experience, taste, hear and feel on a primitive level. Furthermore, what your fetal child feels and perceives in utero begins to shape her attitudes and expectations about herself.

Additionally, her level of activity and the frequency of the activity, as well as her reaction to certain stimulations and events, can tell you a lot about your child's personality. For example, studies show that babies who are very active in utero are more likely to be active babies at ages six months and twelve months.

Another study showed that babies whose heart rate ranged widely with excitement showed similar cardiac variation as a twenty year old adult. As children, these adults tended to be more imaginative and emotional. Try to be aware of the signals your baby is giving you, as well as the signals you are giving to your baby. What is she telling you about herself?

Very likely, your maternal instincts will also have you engaged in nesting activities toward the end of your pregnancy. The heightened anticipation of your baby's birth, and your need to nurture, care for, and protect this child, is then expressed by engaging in such activities. These are natural and instinctual gestures which also begin the early bonding process between you and your baby.

NESTING

What is nesting?

Nesting is the instinctual desire to prepare a space for your baby. It includes buying a crib, changing table, clothing, diapers, etc. You may have a sudden urge to paint or wallpaper the room where your baby will sleep, to clean the garage, or sort the hall closet. These are very natural and instinctive messages that you give to yourself. And undoubtedly, you will experience these urges or desires to one degree or another.

Be cautious. Don't take on too much.

Be very careful about becoming overly zealous about moving furniture, climbing on ladders, and other activities in which you can hurt yourself or the baby. Ask for help. Because I'm very independent, I often thought: "Oh, I can do it myself" during my pregnancies. And usually I could. But I had to remind myself to ask for help with the heavier loads so that I didn't do damage to my unborn babies.

I feel a strong need to buy new baby clothes and furniture. How can I afford to buy all the things my baby will need?

A new layette can be quite expensive when purchased at retail prices. When money is no object, it's easy to buy the newest and finest baby supplies. But when money is an issue, you will have to think creatively to obtain the things your baby will need.

If money is an issue, garage sales, thrift stores, rummage sales, church bazaars and consignment stores are excellent places to go to look for great, affordable bargains. I have found particularly good values in resale consignment shops, which tend to carry more high-end clothing and accessories. When you pick things up second-hand that are new or near new, you will find that the exact same, or like item would cost at least three or four times as much if purchased new.

Talk to your friends who may be able to pass their older baby's newborn clothing or furniture on to you. I have "swap" parties with my friends, where we get together and exchange outgrown clothing and toys with one another. These "swap parties" have proven to be very practical because they don't cost any money, are a good reason for a party, and we all walk away happy with things that we need. I've also found terrific deals on furniture at garage sales and then have refinished or hand painted (non–toxic paint) the items for my childrens' room.

There are organizations, including pregnancy crisis centers that will help out with baby clothing, furniture and formula if your financial situation qualifies you for such services. Further resources can be found at the back of this book.

Tips for buying your layette.

When purchasing new clothing for your baby, unless your child is smaller than average, it is likely that you will find buying clothing in "newborn" sizes to be a waste of money. Buying a few items in newborn sizes is fine, but don't over do it. With shrinkage, and your baby's rapid growth, you will probably find most of the clothing doesn't get much, if any, wear. Buy clothing in small or medium sizes so that your baby can wear the clothing for a longer period of time.

BABY SHOWERS

Wait until after your baby shower to buy for baby.

If you are planning on having a baby shower, it's a good idea to limit what you buy before the shower. This way you can avoid buying two or more of the same item. Showers are usually thrown around the eighth month of pregnancy: so wait to go shopping until you see what your baby still needs once the presents have been opened.

If you don't have someone who has offered to throw you a shower, and you feel uncomfortable asking family or friends to throw one for you, there's nothing wrong with throwing a shower for yourself. This is your special time, and you deserve to have a celebration party. If you feel uncomfortable asking for gifts, let people know how you feel. If you have no problem accepting gifts, by all means, give them directions to your favorite baby store!

You can register at any department or baby store, and then slip a note into the invitation to let your guests know where you're registered. It's a good idea to put inexpensive ticket items along with higher priced items on your registry list. If your friends or family don't have much money, suggest that two or three of them go in on a more expensive item together.

BUDGETING FOR BABY

Lets assume that money does not grow on trees in your back yard. This means that you will need to create a budget for purchasing the items that you did not get at your baby shower.

You will also need money for a variety of other necessary expenses, including, food, diapers, clothing, insurance, doctors, medicines, hair cuts, baby items (crib, car seat, high chair, swing, etc.), lost pacifiers and bottles, child care, recreation, etc., etc. The list goes on and on, and includes surprise and incidental purchases like Christmas and birthday gifts for your child and her friends.

The tangible items you will need to purchase for your baby — above and beyond your own usual monthly expenses — can and may seem overwhelming and burdensome on your budget. Many of you were already stretching your after–tax–dollars to the limit prior to pregnancy or your baby's arrival. The dilemma then, is how to realistically budget for those things that you will need for your baby. The answer is simple and it is not so simple.

Start by making a list.

First, make a list which includes your net (after tax) income and your monthly financial obligations. Then determine what is left over after paying your rent or mortgage, groceries, utilities, etc.

Next, list the items on a priority basis, that are essential purchases for both yourself and your baby on a regular, monthly basis (i.e., food, diapers, medicine, etc.) This list will include items that are non–negotiable — in other words they are *must purchases.*

In another column on your list, list all of the items that are secondary purchases, i.e., clothing, hair cuts, etc. These are items that you can hold–off purchasing over a period of time.

Ideas to help you cut–back on spending.

The idea here is to get a picture of what is essential, what is not, and beyond that, what is possible and practical. Once you have determined your essential monthly obligations (your *must purchases*), you can look at them again to see where you might be able to cut back.

For example, a phone is probably essential, but you can cut down on long distance calls. Gasoline may be essential, but you can cut down on lengthy trips or car pool. Groceries are a necessity, but you can buy store brands and use coupons to save.

Make a grocery list *prior* to going to the store and resist temptation purchases. Consolidate credit cards and use them only when necessary. Those minimum payments might be tempting but interest stacks up and, before you know it, you have paid twice as much for your purchase.

You can also take a bag lunch to work and forego cappuccinos. Use a fan in the summer instead of central air which is more expensive. Find recreational activities that don't cost money. Make gifts for your family and friends for birthdays and holidays instead of purchasing them. Share babysitting and transportation costs with others. And don't forget the fun and value of buying clothing, furniture and other household items at second hand stores or garage sales.

First things first.

There are a multitude of ways that you can cut way back on your usual expenditures after your baby is born so as to accommodate the new monthly necessities you will have to afford. Keep in mind that you do not need to make all of your secondary purchases at once. You can buy them as your finances allow. Of course we always want what we want when we want it. But remember, your baby will be your top priority, not a new haircut, dress, or a more expensive brand of shampoo.

Once you have determined your budget, where you can cut–back and save, and what your actual monthly expenses are, you will then be left with a negative or positive cash flow. Hopefully you will be in the "black". But if you find yourself in the "red", you will need to look at other options which are available to you. You may need to seek some sort of financial aid, including child support from the baby's father. Consider getting a roommate to help cover your rent and utility bills. Such an option can help solve loneliness and babysitting problems as well.

Budgeting for baby when money is an issue is very challenging. I cannot emphasize enough the value of keeping an open mind and being a creative thinker when it comes to seeking solutions to your financial needs. Life will be easier and more enjoyable if you are not constantly worrying about money. So look at all your options, see the possibilities, and be willing to work hard. Your baby's happiness and well–being is worth the price in money and effort.

AFDC/Welfare/food stamps and other programs.

If you find that you are unable to support your child on your own, you may need to turn to government programs for assistance. Depending upon your income, you may qualify for government assistance from any number of programs.

If you qualify, Aid to Families with Dependent Children (AFDC) may be able to assist you with programs, including monthly welfare payments, job training, continuing education, housing, and child care help. Look in your phone book under "Social and Health Services", "Social Services Department", or similar heading in the state government pages of your phone book. Your application will take approximately 30 days to be approved, so be sure to apply well before your baby is due.

If you are not insured, and are having difficulty paying for prenatal care, health care and/or well baby care, you may qualify for Medicaid. Medicaid is a federally funded health program which may pay for your prenatal and childbirth expenses and/or medical coverage for your and your child after his birth. Eligibility is based upon your income. To find out if you qualify for Medicaid coverage, contact your local Medicaid office, listed in the city, state or federal government section of your phone book under "Human Resource Administration", "Social Services Office", or similar heading.

To find out if you qualify for food–stamps, vouchers and other services, call the office of Women, Infants, and Children (WIC), listed under the city, county, or state government section of your phone book, and call your local food stamps office. The food–stamp program is run by the U.S. Department of Agriculture. This program gives free food vouchers to people who work for low wages, receive welfare or other assistance payments, are unemployed, work part–time, are homeless, or are disabled. Even if you have a job, you still may be eligible for this program.

Another organization, Head Start, has over 1,300 centers nationwide offering education and support services for parents, including day care and educational programs for infants from low–income families. For more information call your local public school or Department of Social Services, or look in your phone book under "Head Start Centers."

Welfare Warriors is another organization offering assistance and advice to low–income pregnant women, new mothers, and others receiving government support. A membership in Welfare Warriors costs $15.00 per year ($7.00 for needy women) and includes a subscription to *Welfare Mothers Voice*. For a nominal charge, Welfare Warriors also offers a 185–page *"Mothers' Survival Self–Help Manual"*, which offers information on how to get job training, education, money to support your family, and other issues important to mothers in poverty. To contact Welfare Warriors, call (414) 342–MOMS.

If you can't find the numbers to the government programs listed in this section in your phone book, contact the Federal Information Center at (800) 688–9889. They can provide you with information on all federal programs which may be available to you.

BIRTHING CLASSES

One of the more emotionally difficult things for me to do during both of my pregnancies was to go to prepared child birth classes. Those environments were ones which accentuated my single status more than any of the other situations I encountered.

I attended classes with my sister during my first pregnancy. I was so very glad that she was happy and willing to be my coach, and I was proud to have her be there with me. But I was still a bit daunted by the fact that all the other coaches were fathers. I felt like the odd–woman out because I didn't have a man with me too.

Being a single woman in a couples'–oriented class.

I watched these couples planning the birth of their baby together — observing their interactions, gestures, and expressions toward one another. It all seemed so romantic and larger than life in comparison to my own solo circumstance. Every father in the room appeared to be as excited and emotionally involved as was the mother. These fathers looked tenderly and lovingly into the eyes of their significant other, reassuring these women of their love and devotion to them and their child.

There I sat with my sister, feeling a little jealous and a bit sorry for myself. Where was my significant other! Having one's sister rub one's shoulders, feet, hands, etc., is not the same as having a man do it. And though I was comforted by her presence, and looking into her eyes was nice, it was still a lonely experience for me.

My good friend went with me to classes during my second pregnancy. Though the experience was better that the first time, I still felt somewhat "different", awkward and alone at times. Thankfully, throughout that experience, our teacher was very sympathetic to my single status and refrained from talking too much about daddy's — referring to them as "coaches" instead. That helped a lot.

Sometimes it's hard to stand out in a crowd.

Sometimes it's hard to be the standout in a crowd, especially when one is vulnerable, hormonal — and pregnant. But I was determined to be strong. I reminded myself that being a single–parent was my choice, and that my reward would be holding my child in my arms. With every ounce of courage I could muster during both pregnancies, I went through the first and then the second class with my head held high, and ultimately found the information I gained to be helpful during each of my labors.

If you decide to go to a prepared child birth class, you may find that the "differences" between you and the other coupled students may not present a problem. But be prepared for the fact that you may be the only single–parent in your class. However, because of the rising number of single mothers today, this is beginning to change.

Ask your instructor to be sympathetic to your needs.

If you find that the instructor emphasizes, by choice of words, "daddies", feel free to speak up and tell her that you are sensitive to being without a husband or partner. Ask her to refer generically to "coaches". There is nothing wrong with gently telling someone that your feelings have been hurt and then asking for what you want.

Nonetheless, be prepared for the fact that the focus of the class will be on the mothers' and fathers' roles in the birthing process. The films which are shown will exemplify and portray the loving father's presence in the labor and delivery rooms. Knowing this in advance can help you to prepare yourself emotionally to attend childbirth classes either on your own, or with a friend or family member.

Choosing a partner.

If you will be attending a birthing class with another person, you will need to make sure that this person is willing, ready and able to commit to attending the classes with you, and to coaching you through your labor whenever it begins. Their role in the child's birth is very important, and they should understand exactly what will be expected and required of them.

Be sure that the person you choose is best suited for the job. Don't choose someone because you feel an obligation to them. Often, another woman who has experienced child birth is an excellent choice. She will understand what you are going through, and identify with your labor.

Depending upon the circumstances of your labor and delivery, and the childbirth method you choose, your coach's role may be vital. Under certain circumstances, she or he may need to be assertive on your behalf. Someone who is timid or mild mannered may not be up to the task. So be sure to choose wisely.

You should also know that most obstetric nurses have training in Lamaze or other prepared child birth methods. So it is possible to receive assistance at the hospital from them. However, you can't really count on it because the nurse's schedule may prohibit her or him from giving you the continuous attention you will need during your labor.

If you do not have anybody to go with you to birthing classes or to assist you during your labor, check with your hospital to see what alternatives might be available to you or ask your birth class instructor if she is willing to be your coach. Many instructors do this for a fee.

Hiring a Doula.

Another solution may be to hire a "doula". The word doula comes from ancient Greece, and means 'handmaiden" or "servant". You :an contact the National Association of Postpartum Caregivers at (800) 45–DOULA to see if one is available in your area. A professional doula is an experienced care giver who offers labor support, and also educates and cares for new mothers when they return home from the hospital.

Choosing an appropriate method of childbirth instruction.

There are many different types of prepared child birth classes offered which vary considerably in their approach, methods and ideology about child birth. If you haven't decided what method of childbirth you will use, it's time to consider your options. The following are some of the more popular methods used today:

LAMAZE

The Lamaze method was developed by Dr. Fernand Lamaze in France in the 1940's and 1950's. This method focuses on "mental prevention", and uses special breathing, focus, and relaxation techniques to help a woman's body and mind work together in the birthing process.

Women are conditioned to respond to contractions with "natural and effective" responses, and the coaches are trained to help the mother remember this conditioning — and to facilitate emotional support during labor. Lamaze also provides education on prenatal care and nutritional guidance.

With the Lamaze method, women are not discouraged from using epidural or other forms of medical intervention. For more information on Lamaze classes in your area, call ASPO–Lamaze at (800) 368–4404.

THE BRADLEY METHOD

Founded by Robert Bradley, M.D. and Marjie and Jay Hathaway, the Bradley Method promotes natural child birth where no epidural or other medication is used. It claims a 90% success rate in facilitating unmedicated births. This method emphasizes the coach's role in the birthing process, focuses on education about how your body works during each stage of labor, and discusses the ways which medical interventions may circumvent this natural process. It also emphasizes education on prenatal care and nutritional guidance. For more information on the Bradley Method, and for classes in your area, call (800) 4–A–BIRTH.

THE GAMPER METHOD

The Gamper Method, was named for a nurse who inspired Dr. Grantly Dick–Read, an English obstetrician, who was the pioneer of natural childbirth techniques. The Gamper Method emphasizes education, relaxation, slow abdominal breathing, and caring labor support to combat the three–way cycle of fear, tension, and pain that escalates during labor. For more information, and to find classes in your area, call (312) 248–8100.

Are there other methods available to me?

Yes. Many communities have independent consumer-based education groups that provide classes in childbirth. Look in your local parenting magazine, or in the yellow pages under "Childbirth Education Services" to see what alternatives are available. You can also contact your local hospital to see what classes their maternity section provides.

Whatever class you decide upon, make sure its methods, principles, and practices are in agreement with your own ideas about childbirth. It's important to choose a class that is most representative of the type of labor and delivery you would like to have. Finally, make sure you discuss your choice with your obstetrician so that you work cooperatively in bringing your child into this world.

FEEDING — BREAST OR BOTTLE?

I'm not sure whether I want to breast or bottle feed my baby.

What are your initial feelings about breast–feeding vs. bottle–feeding? Do you feel comfortable with the idea of breast–feeding? If so, you will probably enjoy the close physical relationship that breast–

feeding your baby offers. If, on the other hand, you feel uncomfortable or embarrassed by the idea — the experience may not be enjoyable for you. And if you don't enjoy it, breast–feeding may not work smoothly for you. If you are unsure about what to do, consider what kind of lifestyle you will have after the baby is born.

Will you be staying at home? In this case, either method may suit you. If you return to work soon after the birth, though bottle–feeding may be more convenient, breast–feeding is still possible. However, breast–feeding will require more planning. You will need to make special provisions to express milk for baby to drink while you are away at the office.

Anna, the single mother of a little girl, found pumping breast milk at the office to be easy and convenient — but was embarrassed by the sound her electric pump made behind the closed door of the bathroom stall. Nonetheless, she said it was worth the embarrassment to be able to give her child breast milk. Another mother, Angel, found that she was too stressed at the office to pump milk for her newborn son. She decided that formula was more convenient and gave up breast–feeding altogether.

Whether you choose breast or bottle–feeding, do not allow anyone to pressure you or to criticize your decision. It is your baby, and your body — this decision is yours alone to make.

Making compromises.

With both of my children, I found a workable compromise. For the first few months I breast–fed my babies. When I returned to work, I slowly introduced formula which was intermittently supplemented during the day when I couldn't find the time (often it was too hard on my schedule) to express milk. Finally, by the time I gave up breast–feeding, both of my children were easily switched exclusively to formula.

In my case, I was lucky. Both of my children took the breast or bottle with no problems. However, not all babies make this transition easily.

In order to keep your options open, you will need to start out breast–feeding. You can always change your mind later on and switch to formula. However, you cannot switch from formula to breast. If your baby has not been sucking regularly from your breasts, they will stop producing milk. These factors and considerations will play a role in your decision, but you will also want to look at the facts.

The benefits of breast–feeding.

Pediatricians, obstetricians and even manufacturer's of formulas agree that breast milk is better for your infant than formula for a variety of reasons:

HUMAN BREAST MILK CAN'T BE RECREATED IN A LABORATORY. Breast milk contains at least a hundred ingredients that are not found in cow's milk or formula. Breast milk contains less sodium and protein than cow's milk and thus puts less stress on the kidneys of newborns. Additionally, breast milk contains lower levels of phosphorus. High levels of this mineral can interfere with the utilization of calcium. Cow's milk is tailor–made for calves, not children.

BETTER HEALTH FOR YOUR BABY. Breast milk carries your antibodies which bolster your child's immune system. Babies who are breast–fed tend to come down with fewer colds, respiratory/ ear infections and other illnesses than babies who are bottle–fed.

LOWER RISK OF ALLERGIES. In comparison to formula, breast milk is less likely to cause allergic reactions. Most babies will not be allergic to breast milk. But approximately one in ten will be allergic to cow's milk formula.

BETTER DIGESTIBILITY/LESS RISK OF DIAPER RASH, CONSTIPATION OR DIARRHEA. Breast milk is naturally designed for a newborn's sensitive, developing digestive system. The protein (mostly lactalbumin) and fat content in breast milk are more easily digested than the protein (mostly caseinogen) and fat content found in cow's milk. Evidence indicates that breast–fed infants are less likely to suffer from colic and gas, and tend to do less spitting up. Typically, breast–fed babies have fewer diaper rashes and less incidence of constipation or diarrhea.

LESS EXPENSIVE AND READY TO GO. Breast milk is free (although you may want to invest in a breast pump for expressing milk to store for later use). Formula, on the other hand, will be an added drain on your budget. Furthermore, breast milk needs no preparation, warming up, bottle washing, or storage (unless you want to express milk for later use when you are away from home).

SUPPLY AND DEMAND. Breast–feeding is a natural system of supply and demand. The breasts make milk as your baby drinks. The more he takes, the quicker you will make more. Mother nature has seen to it that your breasts make exactly the right amount of milk to nourish your baby. As he grows, this natural system of supply and demand will cause you to make more to accommodate his growing need for more milk. And you never have to run out to the store to buy more.

FASTER RECOVERY FOR MOM. Breast–feeding helps the uterus return more quickly to its normal, pre–pregnancy size. Another great incentive is that it will help you to burn approximately 500 extra calories per day — which will make it easier to lose those extra pounds and get more quickly back into shape.

BONDING WITH YOUR BABY. There is something very special about the eye–to–eye, skin–to–skin contact breast–feeding affords a mother and her newborn. This is a wonderful way to be closer to your baby.

Breast–feeding and your diet.

If you decide to breast–feed your infant, you will need about 500 calories per day more than your pre–pregnancy intake. These extra calories, in addition to the calories available from the 3–7 pounds you stored in pregnancy for lactation, supply enough calories to make milk. In addition to your intake of extra calories, your breast–feeding diet should include extra protein for milk production. Your diet should contain more calcium–rich foods, more vitamins, and more fluids than your normal diet. The following are simple guidelines you should follow when breast–feeding:

- Unless your doctor tells you otherwise, continue to take your prenatal vitamins.
- Drink more milk than when you were pregnant — about 5 glasses a day. If you have a milk intolerance problem, follow your doctors recommendations to increase your calcium intake.

- Make sure you are drinking plenty of liquids.
- Eat a well–balanced, varied, and healthy diet.
- Avoid junk foods and "empty" calories.
- Stay away from drugs, smoking, alcohol, and caffeine while breast–feeding. These substances can be harmful to your breast–fed baby. Caffeine, alcohol, and drugs pass into breast milk and may cause any number of problems for your baby. Cigarette smoking may also cause complications, including reduced milk production for mother, colicky symptoms and diarrhea for baby. Smoking also decreases the vitamin C content of the milk. Any way you slice the pie, these substances are unhealthy for the breast–fed baby.
- Some of the foods you eat may upset your breast–fed baby's tummy. Some of those foods may include gas producing foods (such as beans, cabbage, and broccoli), eggs, tomatoes, nuts, chocolate, strawberries and other citrus foods, shellfish, corn, onion, garlic, and some spices. If you suspect that a food you are eating is upsetting your baby, you can attempt to isolate the food(s) that bother her by eliminating certain foods (one at a time) from your diet to see if the symptoms disappear.

Is breast–feeding always possible?

No. Some women do not have the option to breast–feed for a variety of reasons, including their health or that of their baby's. You will likely be advised to forego breast–feeding if you have a serious illness such as severe anemia, kidney, heart disease, tuberculosis, AIDS, and possibly hepatitis B. A condition which requires regular medication may also be a factor. Your doctor can discuss these problems with you in more detail and advise you accordingly. Under any circumstances, if you are abusing drugs or alcohol you are not a candidate for breast–feeding.

Another reason a woman may not be able to breast–feed is due to damage to the nerves in the breast (due to injury or surgery). And some doctors recommend against breast–feeding for women who have breast implants — though the data is presently inconclusive. Again, talk to your doctor about these conditions.

Getting started.

For some women, breast–feeding their newborn is awkward or frustrating in the beginning. Nipple soreness, cracking and engorgement (full, rigidly hard breasts) can be very painful, and may discourage many women from continuing.

In some cases, a baby will not "latch–on" to the mother's breast, causing angst for both mother and her hungry baby. But keep in mind that breast–feeding is a learned technique for both mother and baby. Be patient. These problems generally subside within a few weeks or so. Still, many mothers, no matter how prepared or enthusiastic they might have been in the beginning, find the process so discouraging that they abandon their attempts to breast–feed.

If you are having problems with breast–feeding, but want to continue, hang in there. Give yourself enough time to adjust to this new and strange activity. Classes in breast–feeding techniques are available. Organizations such as La Leche League can offer you support in this area. You can contact the La Leche League with breast–feeding questions and concerns at (800) LA–LECHE.

Special problems.

In some cases, a baby may have a lactose intolerance which causes him to be unable to digest breast milk. A deformity such as cleft palate or cleft lip may make suckling impossible. Your doctor will advise you under these circumstances.

If you can't breast–feed, rest assured that commercial formulas, with rare exceptions should be adequate to nourish your baby.

THE OTHER ALTERNATIVE: The benefits of bottle–feeding.

IT'S EASIER TO MONITOR YOUR BABY'S INTAKE.
Many new mothers worry that their breast–fed baby isn't getting enough nourishment. With bottle–fed babies, you can measure the amount of formula your baby receives by looking at the bottle. When breast–feeding, there's no way to determine exactly how much milk your baby gets at one time. A baby who fusses after nursing is probably not getting enough. But if there's no upset, the rate of weight

gain will tell the tale.

DURATION OF SATISFACTION FOR BABY. Formula is less quickly digested than breast milk. The curds formed from cow's milk stay in the baby's stomach for a longer period of time giving the baby a feeling of fullness which can last for several hours. Breast–fed babies digest breast milk more quickly and thus need to be fed more often to feel satisfied.

NO DILEMMAS ABOUT FEEDING IN PUBLIC. Many women are uncomfortable about breast–feeding in public, and some people are uncomfortable about seeing a woman breast–feed in public places. Bottle–feeding means that you will not have to worry about redressing, altering your clothing, (fastening bras, unbuttoning shirts, etc.) and hiding breasts under blankets.

YOUR BREASTS RETURN TO THEIR NORMAL SIZE MORE QUICKLY. You will not need to wear a nursing bra or deal with leaky breasts (especially in public!) And you will be able to wear clothing that is not practical for the breast–feeding mother.

LESS RESTRICTED DIET. When breast–feeding, your diet directly affects your baby. The food you eat is passed on to your baby, and thus spicy, greasy, and other foods may affect your baby's system. The unhealthy foods you eat will also affect your infant. When bottle–feeding, you can eat what you like without having to worry about how it will affect your baby. You can also forego post–natal vitamin supplements, extra protein and calcium. And you can have a few drinks if you like, while the breast–feeding mother is advised to stay away from alcohol. You can also take medications such as anti-biotics and aspirin.

You can begin to diet (but only at least six weeks after your baby is born), whereas dieting *is not* recommended when you are breast–feeding.

MORE CHOICE IN CONTRACEPTIVES. When breast–feeding you are limited to birth control methods that will not hurt your baby. If you happen to have a man in your life, breast–feeding can interfere with sex. Leaky breasts, sore nipples, and dry vaginal area can make sex uncomfortable.

BONDING WITH YOUR BABY. Bottle fed babies bond with their mothers too! You will want to make sure that you take the time to make feedings special. Try not to get into the habit of propping your baby up with a bottle or passing feeding times off to someone else. Take this time to make eye contact, cuddle and hold your baby.

CHOOSING A PEDIATRICIAN

When should I begin to look for a pediatrician?

You should begin to compile a list of potential doctors early in your pregnancy, and schedule appointments to meet with them in your third trimester. Getting an early start on selecting your child's pediatrician will enable you to take your time finding a doctor you trust and like. Realistically, the task of shopping for a doctor during the first few weeks after the birth of your baby will be an exhausting if not impossible task. So it is far better to get this task out of the way in advance of the birth.

Where can I get a list of competent pediatricians to consider?

There are many different ways you can go about finding a good pediatrician. Referrals from friends, family, or co–workers whose opinions you trust is one of the best ways to find a good doctor. Your obstetrician, or primary doctor, can also be an excellent source for recommendations.

If you belong to a PPO or HMO, they may require you to choose from a list of their contracted care providers. But you can still talk with several of the doctors in advance before making a final decision.

Your insurance plan or local hospital will have a referral center which you can contact to request the names of doctors in your area. You can also send a note with your name, address and city or hometown to the American Academy of Pediatrics, Pediatrician Referral, 141 Northwest Point Boulevard, Elk Grove, Illinois 60009–0927 along with a self–addressed, stamped envelope for names of member pediatricians in your area.

If you do not have insurance, contact the Federal Information Center (800) 688–9889. They can provide telephone numbers and information about all federal programs which may be available to you if you qualify. The Hill Burton Hotline (800) 638–0742 can provide information and referrals to local hospital and medical care for low–income women and children. And the National Maternal and Child Health Clearinghouse (703) 821–8955, extension 265 or 254 can provide referrals to local health care providers for you and your child.

How do I narrow down my list of prospective doctors?

First, you should contact the doctors on your list by telephone. Your first impression of the doctor's office starts with the receptionist. Was the phone answered quickly and in a friendly manner? Was the receptionist helpful? Is the doctor available to meet with you for a consultation? Does the doctor charge for consultation services? Does the doctor have any information she can send you describing her practice? Does the doctor contract with your insurance carrier (if that's relevant to your insurance plan)?

Your first impressions are important and say a good deal about the service you will receive from that office. If you like what you hear on the telephone, make an appointment to see the doctor in person. Most doctors allow time in their daily schedules to meet with prospective new patients for a free consultation. Plan to meet with the doctor for about 15-20 minutes. And allow additional time to talk with other patients in the waiting room, as well as with the office staff.

What do I look for when selecting a pediatrician?

Pediatricians vary considerably in terms of philosophies and style. It is important that you select doctor with whom you feel comfortable; someone whom you feel will be responsive to your needs and receptive to your ideas and questions. It is also important that the doctor you choose be supportive of your single–parent status.

When meeting with the doctor, observe his or her mannerisms, voice, smile and body language. These characteristics will tell you a lot about personality and style. Does the doctor seem assertive and formal, or more easy–going and warm? Which style fits best with your needs? Does the doctor answer your questions directly, thoroughly and to the point, in language you can understand?

Observe the atmosphere in the doctor's office. Is there a special area with appropriate materials, games and books for children? Does the office staff seem pleasant and caring? How do they relate to the children waiting to see the doctor? Is the office calm or chaotic? Trust what you feel. Remember, your first impressions are often correct.

Another important factor to consider is the proximity of the office to your home, day care facility, and/or office. Most moms prefer to be within 10-20 minutes of the office.

What are the most important questions I should ask a potential pediatrician?

- How long have you been in practice? What are your affiliations?
- Are you a member of the American Academy of Pediatrics (AAP) or the American Board of Family Practice (ABFP)?
- Do you have one or several locations? How much time do you spend at this location? Who will see my child if you are away from the office? What are your office hours?
- Who will examine my newborn at the hospital? Do you take turns spending time at the hospital with other doctors in your practice? Are you a sole practitioner?
- What is your policy on discharging newborns from the hospital? (24 hours, case by case basis?)
- What are your philosophies on breast–feeding, nutrition (including scheduling and/or introduction to solid foods), vaccinations, (if you do not want to vaccinate your child for example, what are his/her philosophies in this regard), and circumcision?
- Which hospital would you use if my baby needed to be hospitalized?
- When my child is ill, how quickly can I arrange an appointment?
- What training do you require of your telephone nurses and assistants?
- How quickly can I reach you during or after hours in an emer-

gency situation? How long should I expect to wait until I receive a return call after hours? Do you ever make house calls?
- To whom could I direct brief, general questions about my baby's health and other concerns?
- What is the cost of office visits, vaccination, lab work and other necessities? If you do not have health insurance and plan to pay cash, this is a very important factor to consider. Feel free to explain that you do not have health insurance and that fees and costs are an important considerations for you.
- Does the doctor request payment at the time of the visit or will he bill you? Does he offer a package deal for the first year that covers the necessary scheduled visits? Does the office do routine lab work or do they farm it out? (It is usually less costly when done in the office.)

By all means, make a list of these and other questions and take them with you to your consultation visit. Write notes, ask questions, and ask for clarification if you do not understand or are not satisfied with any of the answers you receive.

What happens if I do not select a pediatrician prior to the birth of my baby?

If you do not select a pediatrician for your baby prior to its arrival (one who has privileges at the hospital where you will be delivering your baby), your obstetrician will select a pediatric physician to do a check–up following your baby's birth. The assignment of a physician by your obstetrician at birth will not preclude you from finding your own doctor once you leave the hospital.

WELL BABY EXAMS

Your baby will need to be seen quite frequently during the first three years of life. These visits are important to monitor his growth and development. These visits are also particularly important because *early intervention* can correct problems which, if not treated, can have serious implications for your child later in life.

Your doctor will want to see your baby within 2–3 weeks after his birth, and thereafter at regular intervals. Although most doctors have slightly different scheduled visits, most babies are seen at two, four, six, nine, twelve, fifteen, eighteen, twenty–four, thirty, and thirty–six months old.

During these well baby exams, your doctor will check your baby's ears, nose, throat, eyes, neck, chest, abdomen, hips, genitals, and extremities, among other things to monitor growth and development. Well baby exams are occasions for scheduled vaccinations as well.

Recommended Immunization Schedule

Birth to two months	HB–1 (Hepatitis B)
Two months	HB–2 DTP (Diphtheria, Tetanus, Pertussis) Hib (H, influenza, type b3) TOPV (Polio)
Four months	DTP Hib TOPV
Six months	HB–3 DTP Hib TOPV
Twelve–Eighteen months	DTP Hib MMR (Measles, Mumps, Rubella)
Four to Six years	DTP TOPV MMR (for school admission)

There is a great deal of controversy regarding the need to immunize children. While public health authorities cite the decline in disease occurrence as proof that vaccinations work, critics of immunizations assert that vaccines are capable of causing serious — even fatal — side effects. It is thus important for you to make an informed decision and discuss your concerns with your doctor. In order to make your decision, the following is important: Get information about vaccinations; decide what vaccinations you do or do not want; and if you do decide to vaccinate, choose the right time.

Recommended reading to help you in the decision making process are:

- *The Immunization Decision – A Guide for Parents*, by Randall Neustaedter (North Atlantic Books)
- *Vaccination and Immunisation: Dangers, Delusions and Alternatives (What Every Parent Should Know)*, by Leon Chaitow (The C.W. Daniel Company Ltd)
- *How To Raise a Healthy Child...In Spite of Your Doctor*, by Robert S. Mendelsohn, M.D. (Ballantine Books)

NAMING YOUR BABY

Imagine that your child's name is a colorful ribbon tied in a bow and wrapped around a beautiful gift box. To the receiver, the ribbon is the first impression of the gift inside. In a sense, the name you choose will be the "calling card" of this person you have created, and will help to give your child definition and character. The name you choose will also, to a certain degree, be a reflection of how you picture your baby as a grownup.

Because the name you give to your child will be carried with her through all of the years of her life, great care and consideration should be given to your choice. The opportunity to name your child can be a magical and special event; so allow yourself plenty of time and have fun with the process.

While you may be confused about an appropriate first or middle name for your baby, as a single woman, your baby's last name may offer some additional challenges. Traditionally, married couples give their child the father's last name; so there's usually no question about it. As a single mother, however, you may have concerns over this issue.

Do I have to list the father's name on the birth certificate?

While you are not mandated by law to list your baby's father on your child's birth certificate, you should be aware that not doing so may present future legal issues if a court action ensues. However, many states require a legal paternity affidavit/acknowledgment of paternity, or the father's signature in order to put his name on the birth certificate. You will need to determine the precise requirements of the state in which you reside. Keep in mind, however, that the father's name on the birth certificate does not, in and of itself, establish paternity.

If you list the father's name on the birth record, and he is ultimately ruled out as the child's biological father, with a court order, he can have his name removed from the document.

If I list the father's name on the birth certificate, can my child still use my last name as her legal name in everyday life?

Yes and no — it depends. It is legally okay to do so unless challenged by the father in a court of law and if he prevails on the issue. Oftentimes a mother might choose to list the father's name on the birth certificate — but to use her name for her baby in everyday life. She may feel there will be less confusion, a greater sense of family identity, and perhaps even more social acceptance when she shares the same last name with her child.

However, in some cases, the father in a paternity action may request the court to change the last name of the child to his surname. Because the standard for changing the name is based on "the best interests" of the child, a court may see a name change (to the father's) as being in the child's best interest and grant the change. Fathers can and do prevail in this effort.

I'm not sure how to fill in the line marked "Father" on the birth certificate.

In most states, it is up to you what you fill in on the "father" line. If you do not want to list him on the birth certificate, you can leave the space blank or write "anonymous donor". Keep in mind, however, that your child's birth certificate is a public document, one that you and your child will show to many people over the course of her life. You will want to consider how this may affect her later in life.

Initially, if I use my last name on the birth certificate — but I change my mind later on, can the document then be changed to reflect my child's father's last name?

Yes. The birth record can be changed with a court order. Or, if the father later signs an "Acknowledgment of Paternity", you can send the document to the Registrar Recorders Office to have a corrected version made. While the corrected version will include the father's name, keep in mind that the birth record will then become a two page document. The original remains a part of the permanent record.

Some reasons to give your child his father's last name might be:

- The father intends to play an active and involved role in your child's life; and you plan to co–parent your child with her natural father.
- You eventually seek to establish paternity and an award of child support from the natural father.
- You have strong feelings that the traditional idea of giving a child it's father's last name is appropriate.
- He has a nicer name than you do.

Some reasons you may want to give your child your last name might be:

- Your pregnancy is a result of artificial insemination, or donor sperm.
- Your personal preference is that you and your child share the same last name.
- You do not know who the father is.
- You like your last name better.

Consider your child's particular set of circumstances.

How will your child's last name serve her throughout her life? How will peers, teachers and other adults treat her if her name is different than yours or different than the father's? Although my son Taylor's last name is different than mine, I am often called Mrs. Cross by his teachers and others who assume I must be married to Mr. Cross. Consider the contrasting stigmas for the child: children may ask your child "Why is your name different than your mom's/dad's?"

A compromise –

More and more, we see people hyphenating their last names. These days it is common for a women to use her maiden name in addition to her new husband's (Betty Haley–Carter). Why not consider this option for your child?

When looking at first and middle names, some things you should consider are:

- Is this name one that other kids will make fun of? (i.e., Rusty Nail or Lee King (leaking), etc.
- Does the first and middle name flow with the last name you have decided upon?
- Will the name be easily pronounced or will she have to accentuate it's pronunciation over and over every day of her life?
- What spelling should be given when the name has many different spellings?
- Does the name have an apparent origin or denomination conflict (i.e., Christian Judah)?
- What nicknames will be given to your child. For example, If you have decided upon the name Nicholas, but you do not like the nickname Nick, would that be a problem for you?
- Does the name you give your son or daughter have a "little boy" or "little girl" sound? For example, Bobby, Johnnie, Billy, Becky or Dolly; is that okay for your grown up child?

Think about these things before you make your final decision.

My baby is due this week and I still don't have a name picked out!

Many mothers do not decide until they have given birth or are (literally) about to check out of the hospital. This is a common situation. Many mothers (and fathers) are not sure of a name until the very last moment. Some new parent(s) even leave the hospital prior to giving their baby a name. If a name does not come naturally or easily to you, just know this is not unusual and you are not alone. A decision at the last possible moment, happens all of the time.

Another reason for postponing naming your child until after her birth, may be that meeting your new baby face–to–face, gives you a better sense of her essence. This may inspire you to choose a name that fits your child's being, rather than choosing a name that fits your expectations of who she is before her birth.

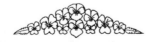

CHAPTER EIGHT

INTO ACTION

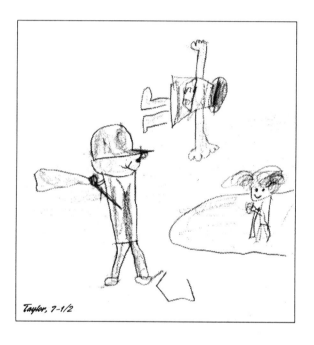

Taylor, 7-1/2

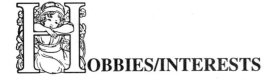OBBIES/INTERESTS

If you do not have a special hobby or interest, get one! I am a painter. I paint functional art (hammers, brooms, mops, screwdrivers, etc.). I also paint furniture. I have spent many lonely and many happy hours painting furniture for my children. (I use non–toxic paint of course). I become so engrossed in my painting that if I felt sad when I started, I forget all about it as my passion for painting consumes me. I also sell my work at a local store which features local artists.

Besides being a passion since I was a little girl, painting is a form of therapy for me. It releases tension and reminds me over and over that I have a special talent. You are good (or great) at something too — or can be with practice.

Finding your special talent.

If you do not already know what you are good at, or what hobby may be fun for you, find out! Start with your interests. What makes you excited? If you're not sure, experiment. If you like nature, start a garden. If you like to cook, become an extraordinary chef. If you're not into stamp collecting, go for something more to your liking — perhaps sewing, reading (positive, uplifting stuff of course!), computers, photography, or bowling (bowling when you are pregnant should be fine if your doctor approves). Try something new. The point is to have interests that keep you balanced, and that help you to take care of your needs for fun, learning, and self–expression.

Engage in hobbies with your child.

For those of you with small children at home, finding hobbies or interests that your child can do with you is especially rewarding and fun for everyone. Inspired by my own love for painting, my son also loves to paint so we do it together often. This activity is relatively inexpensive and is great fun for both of us. Look at your child's interests and your own, and discover something you can come up with that you can enjoy doing together.

GETTING OUT AND GOING PLACES

Do not isolate! Nothing encourages depression, loneliness or sadness like isolation. Abandoning friendships, and foregoing social activities is counterproductive to creating a quality lifestyle. You may have the urge to pull the covers over your head. I certainly have at times. But, for the sake of your emotional health, you can't afford to buy into that. Inactivity breeds inactivity. If you're not feeling very sociable and would rather isolate, don't buy into it! Go out with people anyway!

There will certainly be times when you are tired or "hormonal" and just cannot seem to get it together enough to make plans or keep them. This is to be expected; but don't make a habit of it. If you're having a hard time during your pregnancy, all the more reason you need to focus on having fun. Get out, go places. Meet new people.

Seek out people who help you to feel good about yourself. Whomever you feel comfortable being with, make plans to get together with them. Go to the movies, the beach, museums, to plays or out to dinner. Engage in physical exercise with friends; the buddy system is a great motivator. Get involved in your community. Keeping active, having fun, and enjoying life will enhance your pregnancy and emotional outlook on life.

Make a habit of enjoying activities with your child.

Making a habit of engaging in fun–time activities with your child is important. Your child needs to enjoy quality time with you, engaging in activities that stimulate and excite him. He needs to know that you care enough about him to make the time to share in fun activities. It's important that your child have a very strong sense of family; and family outings promote this bond. The time you dedicate to your child will help build his self–esteem and confidence and will engender trust and friendship between you.

Although you may be very busy with work and other chores, it is imperative that you set time aside each week to get out and have "kid–fun." Take your child to the park. Fly kites or play hide–and–seek. Go to the beach, a children's museum, the zoo, the library, observatory, etc. Have a picnic, take walks together, or go hiking. Get your child involved in a "play group" with other children. Look in the calendar section of your local newspaper to find activities that you can share with your child.

There are so many things you can find to do; and many won't cost you a dime. Kids need to get out and go places. Staying in the house all cooped up is not exactly their idea of a good time. Have fun, get out, and enjoy yourself and your child.

POSITIVE PEOPLE

Have you ever noticed when a person who is negative or angry walks into a room, your own energy is affected? Perhaps you have a friend who is constantly depressed, or a friend who takes unfair advantage of you. Do you find yourself absorbing their energy and becoming uncomfortable when you are with him or her? We can be magnets for other people's negative energies, particularly when we ourselves are vulnerable.

Don't borrow trouble.

If you are borrowing trouble by aligning yourself with people who are negative and do not support your emotional fulfillment, it's time to look at your reasons why you are attracted to them. What are you getting out of relationships that do not support your growth and development?

It is unfortunate, but sometimes the people we attract into our lives cause us tremendous pain. Though we may know they do not contribute to our happiness, we continue to keep them in our lives anyway. We complain about them, and yet we do nothing to change the situation — at least not until things finally erupt and explode. Why do we do this? Why are we attracted to "lower companions" or negative people? What are we getting out of these relationships?

Pop–psychology tells us that we are attracted to such people because we are living out unresolved relationships from our past. Familiarity, for many of us, is "comfortable" — *even* if it is painful and unhealthy for us. Many of us believe (consciously or subconsciously) that we don't deserve happiness; and thus we are attracted to those who do not encourage it.

It's time for a change — making better choices.

Whatever the reason, if you are aligning yourself with people who are not encouraging your happiness and unfoldment, it's time for you to make a change. You are worthy of relationships that encourage, not discourage your emotional well–being.

Because your happiness, self–esteem, and fulfillment are affected by the company you keep, make a conscious effort to attract people who are uplifting, bright, positive and cheerful. Choosing friends with these qualities will have a positive effect upon you. People who are supportive and treat you with respect, are the people you want to attract into your life.

Your child will model your behavior.

Positive relationships are also reflected in our children's hearts and minds. If our children see us choosing and modeling positive relationships, they will be more likely to choose positive relationships for themselves. If we are stuck in relationships that are negative or destructive, our children will think that these are normal conditions. They will accept them as being okay.

But they are not okay, and they are not healthy. It is important that you surround your child with as much positive energy as possible. Positive relationships will reflect in his attitude and outlook on life.

Try to pay attention to the kind of energy and emotions you are displaying toward and around your children as well. Your own negative energies and emotions will affect him significantly. Your child will surely pick up on, and become influenced by them.

Presumably, you want your child to be a positive and bright individual with a cheerful disposition. By exposing him to positive people, yourself included, you can help guide him to fulfill those desires.

WHEN YOU'RE DOWN... HELP OTHERS LESS FORTUNATE THAN YOURSELF

In those times when I am hurt or deeply distressed, an amazing transformation occurs in my heart and mind when I help someone less fortunate than myself. Giving freely of myself is truly meaningful and important to my healing. When I can stop feeling sorry for myself long enough to help someone else, the joy I receive is one of the greatest gifts I can give to myself. Charity, when given from the heart, is among the most miraculous healing and loving expressions I have known. Giving to others gives my own life deeper, richer meaning.

Lets face it, being pregnant, and being a single parent is sometimes very difficult. There may be times when you are feeling sorrier for yourself than is good for you. When you look to the horizon and see only difficulty and despair, this is the time to get into action! Getting out of yourself and giving to another is a wonderful way to heal and to regain hope and encouragement in your own life. When you view life through the eyes of someone who has greater challenges than you, often your perspective will change about your own situation.

For me, it is easy to be selfish; and it is also so easy to be selfless and giving. This is my choice to make. But because I want my children to have a deep appreciation for other people and to understand what giving is all about, I attempt to model charitable behaviors for their benefit. I want my children to grow up to be caring and compassionate human beings, concerned about others. I must therefore set an example so they will follow and grow to be caring, giving adults.

We can do big or small deeds. Perhaps donating time to a worthy organization or hospital; giving $5.00 to a good cause when we've only got $20 to spare; helping a friend in need; answering a hotline, etc. How about going with your children to a homeless shelter to give their old toys and clothes to needy children? There is much to be done. It doesn't matter what our deed, as long as our gestures are sincere and intended to benefit someone else. In doing so, the gift we receive in our hearts in return is far greater than what it cost us to give.

CHAPTER NINE

EVERYDAY LIFE – COMMON CONCERNS

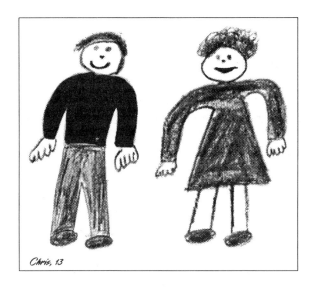

Chris, 13

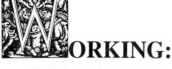

ORKING:
DURING AND AFTER PREGNANCY

Unless you have other sources of income, or you are independently wealthy, it is likely that you will need to work during your pregnancy and perhaps after. Working may be a preference, or it may be a necessity. In either case, there are many details pertaining to your job/pregnancy which need to be worked out prior to your baby's arrival.

Taking care of yourself on the job.

Depending upon the type of job you have, and the way your pregnancy is progressing, it may be possible for you to work up until the end of your pregnancy. There are, however, precautions you should take if you are working:

- Take frequent breaks. If you are in a sedentary position for long periods of time, stand up and walk around; at least every hour, but every half hour is better. Do some stationary stretching exercises to help circulation.
- If you sit for long periods of time, keep your legs elevated (on a stool, etc.) if possible. Make sure your chair offers adequate support and a firm cushion to help eliminate stress on your back.
- If you are standing for long periods of time, keep one foot on a low stool, with your knee bent. This will help prevent the strain on your lower back. When standing on a hard–surfaced floor, a small rug will help to cushion the pressure on your back. Ask your doctor about the benefits of a pregnancy girdle or support sling for your belly. It may lessen the stress on your lower back. Wearing support hose is also helpful.
- Cut down on strenuous activities (both on and off the job). If you are feeling tired, take it easy. Listen to what your body is telling you. Take a nap whenever necessary and possible.

- Never do heavy, abrupt lifting. Lifting weights of about 25 pounds on a consistent basis should not be a problem; and up to 50 pounds intermittently — up to approximately the twentieth week. If you do lift heavy loads on the job, or lift children, groceries, packages, etc., lift with your arms, not your back. Always bend at the knees, not at the waist.
- Wear shoes with proper support. Stay away from high heels. Your feet may swell as your pregnancy progresses. Invest in a good pair of shoes for optimal comfort.
- Stay away from smoke–filled rooms. The smoke can increase your fatigue, and is not healthy for you or your baby.
- Avoid extremes in temperatures.

Talk to your doctor about what restrictions, if any, you should follow on the job. Let your doctor know what your job entails, as many occupations are potentially hazardous to you and your fetus. If your job is hazardous, or you work with toxic, noxious fumes, consult with your doctor. Ask your employer if there is an another department you can transfer to during your pregnancy. Your doctor will determine how long you can stay on the job. Always defer to his or her instructions.

Making the announcement of your pregnancy to your employer.

It's usually a good idea to hold–off telling your boss or supervisor about your pregnancy until after your first trimester. By waiting until you are well into your second trimester (about the fifth month), you may avoid several months of awkwardness, or unpleasant reactions from your employer and co–workers. You will also have the opportunity to prove your ability to deal effectively with your job and your pregnancy simultaneously.

If you hold–off telling your employer, however, it's a good idea to hold–off telling your co–workers as well. News travels fast. Even if your friends or co-workers are sworn to secrecy, your boss may find out anyway. The news of your pregnancy is much better coming straight from you.

When you're ready to sit down with your boss and talk about

your pregnancy, make an appointment to meet with him or her in private. Be prepared for any number of reactions. Your employer may be fully supportive, or feel threatened by the news. There's no way to tell how your boss will respond.

If your employer does not take the news well, you should be aware that the law stipulates that pregnancy alone is not grounds for an employer to dismiss an employee as long as she is able to work. Nonetheless, many women experience harassment in the workplace after disclosing they are pregnant — either subtle or blatant harassment.

Discrimination in the workplace.

Many women find they are subjected to discrimination and criticism or are patronized in the workplace by employers and co–workers alike. In some cases women have been fired, demoted (or hidden away once they start to show). They've been passed over for promotions, had work schedules arbitrarily rearranged, had workloads shifted away from them to others, etc.

If you feel you are being harassed, be sure to make notes pertaining to the incident(s), including time, date and person(s) involved, and write down names of any witnesses. It's also a good idea to keep a record of your attendance, job performance, and any other pertinent information. This information will help if you find you need to take steps, legal or otherwise, to correct the problem.

The Pregnancy Discrimination Act.

In 1978 the U.S. Congress passed the Pregnancy Discrimination Act which provides that employers must treat pregnancy as other temporary disabilities are treated. In other words, you are entitled to the same benefits as other employees in your company would receive if they were to become temporarily disabled by reason of illness or accident.

If you have been fired or otherwise discriminated against, after you have exhausted all efforts to resolve the matter on your own, call the U.S. Equal Employment Opportunities Commission at (800) 669–EEOC, or the Department of Labor, Women's Bureau Clearinghouse

(800) 827–5335 for advice and assistance. If you decide to file a complaint, be aware that you must file a complaint within a certain period of time after the incident occurred (usually several months), so be sure to report the problem immediately.

The Family Medical Leave Act of 1993.

Under the Family Medical Leave Act of 1993, if your company employs at least 50 people, you may qualify for 12 weeks of unpaid leave in any 12 month period. However, some states require companies to provide more than the 12 weeks mandated by the federal government. Such unpaid leave can be for the birth or adoption of a child, to care for your child, spouse or parent with a serious health condition, or for your own serious health condition which makes it impossible for you to perform your job. Some guidelines regarding this Act are as follows:

- Any company with fewer than 50 employees is exempt.
- Your employer can deny leave to you if you are among the highest paid 10% of its work force *and* if letting you take a leave of absence would create "substantial and grievous in-jury" to business operations.
- Your employer may require medical opinions and certification confirming the need for a leave of absence.
- Your employer must return you to your old job, or an equivalent position upon your return to work.
- In order for you to qualify for this leave of absence, you must have been employed for at least one year *and* for an average of at least 25 hours per week for the prior year (1,250 hours).
- You cannot collect unemployment or other government compensation while on this type of leave. (This will make it hard for many to take advantage of such a leave of absence.)
- If your employer provided you with health care benefits prior to your leave, your employer must maintain the policy during your leave as if you were still employed. *However*, your employer is not obligated to pay the premiums during your leave.
- If your employer paid your health care premiums, and you later decide not to return to work, your employer may seek reimbursement from you for all premiums paid by it.

For additional information about the Family Medical Leave Act, contact the Department of Labor's Women's Bureau Clearinghouse, or "9 to 5," a national working women's advocacy group, at (800) 522–0925.

Other considerations to discuss with your employer:

- Does your employer offer paid maternity benefits. If so, how long? Will you receive full pay, or a portion thereof?
- When will your maternity leave begin, and when will you be expected to return to work?
- How will your job be handled in your absence?
- Does your company offer flex–time (job sharing with another person on a part time basis?) This can be a beneficial situation both during pregnancy and after your baby is born.
- Does your employer offer on–site day care? (Larger corporations often offer this benefit).

If your employer does not offer paid maternity leave, you may be eligible for disability benefits.

Unfortunately, some employers are unable to offer sick leave or disability benefits to any of their employees. If you are not paid for your maternity leave by your employer (or if you are only paid a portion of your normal salary), you should check with your state's Employment Development Department, (or it's equivalent agency), to determine whether you are eligible for disability benefits during your maternity leave.

Note: your employer can count any paid leave under your disability coverage as part of your 12 weeks unpaid leave mandated by the Family Medical Leave Act.

Working mothers.

Being a full–time working mother is definitely a challenge, particularly when you don't have help. Unfortunately, economics often dictate that you work at a full–time job. And sometimes trying to do it all feels like spinning plates: you run from one to the next because if you stop, they all come crashing down around you. Then you wake up the next day and do it all over again.

However, with the right attitude, and by employing constructive time management, you can do a very good job meeting your responsibilities. But you will need to be very creative to most effectively meet the demanding needs of your job, baby, housework, personal life (yes, you can have one), doctors appointments, illnesses, school activities, among the countless other things that can, and will come up. But you can do it! Remember that the tools of affirmations, meditation, visualization, exercise, writing, etc. can be used whenever life or career become overwhelming.

The need or the choice to work does not mean that we cannot be good parents; and it certainly doesn't mean that we don't love our children just as much as stay–at–home moms.

HOUSING

If finances are a problem for you and you cannot afford to live where you like, you may need to get creative with solutions to this dilemma.

If you live in a small apartment — though you may wish to get a bigger place to live — your apartment can work out just fine. Sharing a room with your baby is most often more convenient for new mothers anyway. If you have a one bedroom apartment, perhaps you can turn a large closet or dining area into a second room for your baby or small child. For some, a roommate (perhaps another single mother) works out great. Still, for others, moving in with family or other relatives is a workable solution.

If you are having problems locating affordable housing, contact your local Low–Income Housing office listed under Housing Assistance in the government pages of your local directory. You can also contact the Department of Housing and Urban Development, at (202) 708–2495 for information on low–income housing in your area. Finally, if your income is low–to–moderate, and you want to purchase your own home, contact ACORN (202) 547–9292 for help in applying for and getting a loan.

DATING – DURING AND AFTER PREGNANCY

Do men find pregnant women attractive? And do women actually date during pregnancy?

It is not at all uncommon for some men to be attracted to pregnant women; finding them to be very sensual, sexy and appealing. If you are feeling emotionally prepared to date while you are pregnant and you meet an interesting man who is not intimidated or daunted by your situation, by all means, go out with him!

Dating can be a lot of fun, and male companionship can be very uplifting and healthy for you. There are undoubtedly those of you who will say "I can't date, I'm pregnant!" Perhaps you are not yet over *him*, or the idea of dating at this time in your life is simply not desirable to you. That's fine. If you are not interested in dating, then don't give it another thought.

However, there's nothing wrong with doing so if the opportunity arises. I know several women who dated when they were pregnant and ended up marrying the man (not the father of their baby). These men are now raising the children as their own.

A word of caution: You are apt to be more vulnerable during pregnancy, and the desire to be with someone who will take care of you may be stronger than usual. While this is not necessarily a bad thing, be careful not to get involved with someone for the *wrong* reasons. Don't settle for less than you deserve, and don't use a man out of selfishness.

Dating and the single mother.

When you are a single–parent and you are thinking it's about time for you to get out and begin dating (if you have not already been doing so), you obviously will have other concerns relating to your situation, especially as dating affects or concerns your baby or young child(ren). Introducing your child to the men you are dating, child care, self–esteem issues, etc. will certainly be factors and reasons to consider what is or is not appropriate for you.

I found that it was comfortable for me to start dating just before my son, Taylor turned one. And though I did not choose to date during either of my pregnancies, I did go out and have fun with male friends.

When I did ultimately begin to date, it served as an important reminder that I was not just "Mommy", but that I am a desirable, interesting woman. However, I found that some men cannot handle the fact that I have children. I decided that if a man doesn't intuitively and naturally like kids, then he is not for me anyway.

Some men don't relate well to children.

If you've decided to date, and eventually you decide to introduce your child to the man you're interested in, observe how he relates to your child. A pat on the head and saying something detached like "Nice little boy" won't do! It is important that a man have a genuine interest in children and be comfortable around them.

Surprisingly, many men will date a woman whom they find interesting and wonderful. But they do not want to have anything to do with her child. They feel that if the kid would just somehow disappear, everything would be fine. In the long run, this situation will only lead to disappointment. A man must accept you and your child as a package deal. There is no negotiation on this point.

It's not healthy to live in a vacuum.

Don't cut off a social life because you feel you are protecting your child from exposure to such a lifestyle. It's not healthy for you and it's not healthy for your child to live in a vacuum. Besides, your child learns from what he sees you do. If he sees you having a good time enjoying a healthy relationship with one special, loving partner, he will be more likely to model such behavior in his own life. Dating is part of being single and having fun. Just use your best judgments about safety and exposure.

Taking precautions.

When dating, I have found it best not to let a man pick me up at my house or even meet my children until I have been dating him for a little while, both for safety reasons as well as to protect my children from virtual strangers.

I prefer to meet a man at a restaurant or an open, well lit, crowded place. I do not want my kids to have transient male figures running in and out of their lives. And frankly, I'm not sure until I know a man fairly well if he is good enough to meet my kids. So I find it is better to exercise discretion for my sons' and my own sake.

It is important to protect our children from a revolving door of men. While dating is fun and important, a flow of men who come and go can harm our children in many ways. Self esteem may suffer: "Every man leaves me eventually — just like Daddy". Or, a child may see himself as the cause for men leaving.

He may be angry at you for betraying his father. He may feel threatened that *you* will leave him if you fall in love with someone else. He may worry that a man will take your time away from him. Our children will have any number of feelings about our dating — from positive to negative — depending upon the circumstances and the child.

While I am not a mother who believes a woman should keep her social life completely hidden from her child or children, single mothers need to be particularly careful in this area. Sensitivity toward your child's feelings is critical. At the same time, it is very important for your child to understand that Mommy is a separate individual from him, who likes to have time to herself to date and do grown-up things.

Your child needs to know that he must share Mommy with her work and a social life. It is, however, so important to use precaution and discretion when you are dating. Be sure that you are spending enough one-on-one time alone with your child, and keep the lines of communication open.

Introducing your child to a man you are dating.

If you decide to introduce your child to someone you've been dating, take care to introduce them to one another in a casual and comfortable setting. If your child is old enough, talk with her beforehand about her feelings concerning your dating. Her feelings are very important and she should feel free to express them to you.

You may have some rough spots to get over in this area. The

dating game is not always smooth or easy for you or your child. In fact, it can be frustrating and draining — on both of you.

Including your child on a date.

Once you've decided to introduce your child to a terrific man, including your child on a date can be a lot of fun for everyone. When making the date, choose a relaxed setting where everyone will be comfortable.

One time I decided it would be nice for my son, Taylor to meet a man I was dating. To make Taylor comfortable, we all went to Chucke Cheese's, a child–oriented pizza parlor. It turned out to be a very good idea. It was relaxing and enjoyable and there was no pressure on any of us. Taylor had built–in fun and could come and go from our table as he pleased. I had fun and the fellow had fun (he had never been to a theme pizza parlor and thought it was great). I was able to have some grown–up conversation at the same time that I was enjoying my son and his fun–time activities.

Judgment from men about single mothers.

Catherine, a single mother of a five year old, recounted to me the story of a man who was interested in dating her — until he found out she was a single mother. When he found out she had a baby without being married to the child's father, he asked her how this "happened to her" because she "seemed like such an intelligent woman".

His message was pretty clear: he didn't approve. Catherine went on to say that, from time to time, she was asked similar questions by other people as well. Often the tone of their voice, and the slant of their questions seemed to her to denote contempt or disapproval of her and her circumstances.

While many of the mothers I interviewed had experienced such situations, happily, many others had not. Alison, a divorced, single mother of a vivacious three year old, has never experienced any prejudice or inappropriate questions asked of her about her situation. And Sherry, a single mother of two children from two different fathers, reports that she has only experienced support and kindness toward her and her children from the men she dated and from others in her community.

Every woman will experience different reactions and find different levels of support, or lack of support, from the people in her community, church, family and friends.

For me, it has cut both ways. I have been asked numerous personal questions over the years..."You mean you didn't marry your baby's father!", or even more direct, "Do you think it's fair for you to raise your children without a father?" These are just a few of the many questions people have asked me. Such questions can be annoying and even hurtful, but people ask them anyway.

On the other hand, I have received more overwhelming support and praise for the job I do with my kids. People will often say "Wow — what a great job you do!" In particular, many men whom I have dated over the years offer encouragement and praise for the job I do. It's wonderful to receive the acknowledgment.

SEX AND MASTURBATION DURING AND AFTER PREGNANCY

If you do not have a significant other in your life, sex will likely not be an issue for you. However, some of you may still be tied in some way to the baby's father, to an old boyfriend or a fellow with whom you get together every now and then for company and/or sex. This is a touchy subject for some, but is a reality for others.

Your sex drive during pregnancy.

You may find that you do not have the same sex drive as you did before you were pregnant. In fact, sex may be a total turn-off. Or, you may find your interest in sex has stayed the same or even greatly increased during pregnancy. It can be a confusing time for many pregnant women.

You may have been very interested in sex prior to pregnancy, and now you have no sexual desire to speak of — and visa versa. Where no sex drive was apparent before pregnancy, you now have a voracious appetite for sex. Further, some women who never had an orgasm before may experience orgasms — even multiple orgasms during pregnancy. Every pregnancy is different and every woman's sexual needs are different. All are perfectly normal.

Sex during pregnancy.

I would definitely not suggest that you go out and find a sex partner while you are pregnant. But if you have already been seeing someone and are interested in having sex, doctors tell us that if your pregnancy is progressing normally, you have no vaginal discharge or bleeding, and you are comfortable about having sex then it is fine to do so. To be safe, ask your doctor about his or her recommendations regarding sex during your pregnancy.

Common concerns regarding sex during pregnancy.

You will likely have concerns about having sex during your pregnancy. The following will help you to alleviate fears and understand sexuality during pregnancy:

- **Breast tenderness:** Your breasts may be highly sensitive or painful during pregnancy. Tenderness should diminish toward the end of your first trimester. For some women, the increased sensitivity can enhance sexual experiences. If your breasts are painfully tender, be sure to communicate this to your partner. Don't suffer through needless pain in silence.
- **Vaginal secretions:** Whitish vaginal secretions (leukorrhea) increase in volume, change in consistency, odor and taste. You may find that lubrication is increased or diminished. If lubrication is diminished, you may need to use a lubricant. Be sure to ask your doctor before using any lubrication remedies.
- **Vaginal bleeding:** During pregnancy, the uterus becomes engorged and softer. This, coupled with the additional blood vessels developed to accommodate increased blood flow to the uterus occasionally results in bleeding after deep penetration, particularly in late pregnancy. If this occurs, let your doctor know just to be on the safe side.
- **Your ever–growing figure.** As your pregnancy progresseyou may find that sex causes you to feel physically and emotionally awkward or uncomfortable. You may need to alter and ex-

periment with your usual positions for comfort, and to make room for your new and expanding figure. Being pregnant does not mean being unattractive. Your acceptance of your beauty and belly will go a long way toward more satisfying, passionate lovemaking.

- **Those leaky breasts.** During the mid–to–latter part of your pregnancy, your breasts may begin to produce premilk called colostrum. When you become sexually stimulated, you may find that your breasts leak. If this occurs, and it causes you or your partner to become uncomfortable, the only way to avoid discomfort is to avoid breast play.

- **Concern that an orgasm will cause miscarriage or early labor:** The uterus contracts following an orgasm, and for some women, these contractions can be quite pronounced. For some, contractions can last for a half an hour or longer after an orgasm. In a normal pregnancy, such contractions are not an indication of labor. However, if you have a high–risk pregnancy, your doctor will likely tell you to refrain from intercourse and/ or masturbation.

- **Concern that intercourse will harm your fetus**. If your pregnancy is progressing normally, intercourse will not harm your baby. The fetus is protected inside the amniotic sac and uterus; further cushioned by the mucous plug in the mouth of the cervix. Although fetal reactions during intercourse indicate slowed movement, followed by elevated heartbeat, squirming and kicking after orgasms, these are reactions to the hormonal and uterine activity, and not to the intercourse. Your baby will be fine and may actually enjoy the gentle rocking of uterine contractions.

  In the latter stages of your pregnancy, you may fear that during intercourse the penis will "hit" the baby's head. Though this does not occur, most doctors suggest that deep penetration should be avoided.

- **Knowing when to stop having intercourse.** Generally, unless you have a history of miscarriage, or show signs of a miscarriage, you can enjoy sex into the ninth month; although some doctors suggest you refrain from sex four to six weeks before delivery. Your doctor can advise you best on this matter — be sure to ask. Don't be embarrassed to talk candidly and openly with him or her.

Practice safer sex under *any* circumstances.

You should, of course, take appropriate precautions to protect yourself against disease and infections by utilizing condoms — both during and after pregnancy. Safer sex is very important. If you contract a disease or infection, this could well be very dangerous or even detrimental to you and to your unborn baby. Of course, no sex is the only safe sex.

After the birth of your baby, if you don't want to become pregnant again, don't play Russian Roulette with your body. If you are sexually active, talk with your doctor about birth control. *Note:* it is a myth that you cannot become pregnant while breast–feeding — you can!

Masturbation.

If you do not have a sexual partner, and you feel the need for sexual fulfillment during your pregnancy, it is perfectly healthy, natural and normal to pleasure yourself by masturbating. Masturbation is harmless to you and your fetus, unless you are experiencing complications during your pregnancy. In fact, orgasms are terrific in helping to relieve stress, relax you, and fulfill your sexual tensions.

Sex and the single mother.

When you have young children, your sexual relations, at least in your own home, should be discreet and private. You will need to exercise good judgment about where and when to engage in relations with a man, especially one whom your child does not know. Having a child in the home should not preclude you from engaging in safe sex if you so choose. However, using common sense and considering the needs of your child is essential.

Having multiple sex partners is clearly detrimental to the family structure — and to you as an individual. A child should never be exposed to a flow of strangers coming out of Mommy's bedroom.

This will undoubtedly cause confusion and fear. As they grow, children will form definite opinions about this type of indiscriminate behavior. They may rebel, or ultimately copy the behavior.

In any case, when a child is old enough, they will figure out what is going on and it will leave a lasting impression. Displaying responsible behavior is important. As parents, we must respect ourselves in order to teach respect.

Finding a balance between your needs and those of your child can sometimes be difficult when it comes to this issue. Age–appropriate communication with your child is essential to maintaining your healthy relationship with her. And using common sense, good judgment, and putting your child first will help to eliminate unnecessary problems with respect to the issue of your sex life.

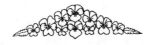

CHAPTER TEN

THE REALITIES OF MOTHERHOOD

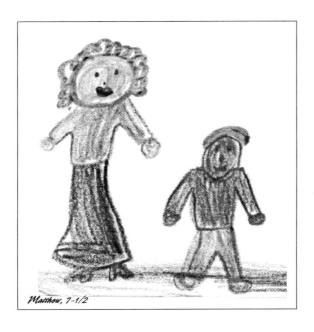

Matthew, 7-1/2

BONDING WITH YOUR NEWBORN

The interaction which takes place between you and your new-born infant directly after birth will serve to enhance the bond between you. This interaction continues the process of bonding which began during your pregnancy. Your attachment to your new baby literally serves to ensure her care and thereby her survival.

Many new mothers have an intense need to be near their babies after they are born. Fortunately, most hospitals have rooming in, and barring any complications, your baby should be able to stay with you in your room.

After your baby is born, you will probably want to explore her by stroking her face, arms, and legs, and by counting toes and fingers. Your instinct to breast–feed your baby (if it is your intention to do so) may also begin shortly after she is born.

Studies have indicated that although a bond can be formed later (if, for example, a baby is taken away from it's mother immediately), the best time for the attachment to form is during the "maternal sensitive period" which is directly after birth.

Based upon our current understanding of the bonding process between a mother and her newborn infant, the optimal conditions for each is when the mother and baby are healthy and alert following delivery; neither has been drugged; the baby has suffered no oxygen deprivation during the birthing process; the lights in the room are dim; and the newborn is placed immediately upon the mother, even prior to the umbilical cord being cut. These are circumstances that will facilitate the bonding process.

I don't feel the wild euphoria toward my newborn that so many new mothers talk about. Is there something wrong with me?

Although many mothers begin bonding with their child while they are pregnant and immediately after the birth, this is not always the case. In fact, not every mother falls in love with her child either during pregnancy or immediately after the baby's birth. What most baby books, magazine articles, doctors, and other mothers don't tell us is that some of us take a little longer to "fall in love" with our babies. A delayed bond is also natural and considered normal; we just don't hear women running around saying "I looked at my new baby and didn't feel a rush of love and emotion at first — it took awhile."

I'm not sure why women tend not to talk openly about this experience. But I think it may have something to do with shame or feelings of inadequacy.

The fact that it takes some of us longer to bond with our new baby does not make us any less loving, equipped, or ready to be a mother. Simply, each of us is different, and our experiences will differ. So too will our attachments to our child. Bonding will occur in its own good time; and not necessarily at the hospital or right away.

Every pregnancy, labor and delivery is different for each woman, and circumstances at home and in the personal lives of individual will be different. All of these factors play a contributing role in the bonding process between mother and child. The more stress–free, emotionally and physically healthy the mother is, the better the attachment to the baby will be.

THE "BLUES"

Roughly one–half (though some estimates go as high as 90%) of new mothers experience the "blues" during the first week or so after delivery. The blues may include bouts of crying, unhappiness, mood swings, and anxiety.

The condition is probably related to the sudden drop in estrogen and progesterone after childbirth, and usually clears up within a few days — although some new mothers find that it comes and goes for a period of as long as six weeks.

POSTPARTUM DEPRESSION

Postpartum depression is different than the "blues". It often begins during the first six weeks, and can persist for a much longer period of time; sometimes even months.

What causes postpartum depression?

Medical experts have not been able to agree on the exact cause of this depression. Some experts contend that the sudden drop in the level of maternal hormones causes this problem. Others believe the depression can be related to a complicated birth with prolonged labor. There are those who believe that the separation of mother and baby at the hospital causes the depression. There are so many opinions, but no real evidence that one situation over another causes or contributes to this problem.

Signs and symptoms of postpartum depression.

Some of the symptoms of postpartum depression are crying for no apparent reason, anger, anxiety, severe mood swings, helplessness, numbness, feeling detached from your baby — or overconcern for her, feeling inadequate, erratic sleep patterns, thoughts of suicide, headaches, lack of physical energy, confusion, worry, or lack of appetite.

Contributing factors.

There are many other factors which are believed to contribute to this problem. Some of these non–hormonal factors may explain why fathers and adoptive mothers who have no hormonal changes also experience this depression.

Some factors may include:

The end of the pregnancy. There may be a sense of loss or emptiness after the birth of your baby. You may miss the sensation of carrying your baby — and even regret the disappearance of your bulging stomach. You may experience an anticlimactic feeling. The big event of childbirth has come — and gone.

Going home. It can be overwhelming — especially for single mothers — to return home to so many new responsibilities. Dirty laundry, dirty dishes, and other chores can be difficult to deal with when you have no help — as can this demanding new creature who has come to live with you.

Exhaustion/loss of sleep. Fatigue, following your child's birth, coupled with the responsibilities of caring for your newborn, can make these early days and months very difficult. You might even feel unable to meet the numerous challenges you face. Loss of sleep won't help much either. Sleep deprivation causes mood swings, and can induce postpartum depression.

Loss of attention. Your new baby now receives all of the attention. Both at the hospital, and after you go home, people are now more interested in your baby than they are in you. All of the attention you received during pregnancy has vanished.

Disappointment. Motherhood may not be all you expected it to be. Perhaps the birth process didn't go smoothly; or your baby just isn't quite the personality you expected. You may feel this isn't what it was cracked up to be. Maybe you wanted a boy and got a girl. And the reality that life has changed for good and that this child is for keeps can be truly daunting.

Discomfort or physical pain. It's hard to feel good when you are in physical discomfort. Episiotomy or cesarean incision pains, engorged breasts, after–pains (uterus contractions), or hemorrhoids may contribute to depression.

Lack of support/stress. If you don't have enough support around you — from friends and family — the job of mothering may seem depressing and overwhelming. And missing *him* may trigger resentments, pain or sorrow. With so much going on right now, you are feeling pushed to the limit. This results in stress, which can contribute to postpartum depression.

Feelings of guilt, resentment, or inadequacy. New mothers go through a gambit of emotions. You may feel guilty about any number of things. Not having a father for your child — or maybe you didn't want her at first. You may be angry at her for how she has changed your life — or blame her for her father going away. You may feel a complete inability to properly care for this child, and doubt your abilities to deal with her. Such emotions can easily bring on depression — whether they are unfounded or natural feelings and emotions.

Feeling Ugly or Fat. This baby has stretched your body to the limits. Your skin may be dry, and your hair — well, you don't even recognize it anymore. You're tired of wearing maternity clothes, and you just feel fat.

Diet. With all of your new–found responsibilities, you may be missing the proper nutrition you need right now. An insufficient diet can help trigger depression.

Does every new mother experience postpartum depression?

No. Approximately 50% of new mothers describe the feelings they experienced after the birth of their baby as euphoric and uplifted. They show no signs of postpartum depression. The other 50% experience this depression to varying degrees — from slight to severe.

What can I do to combat postpartum depression?

Try to accept that your depression exists, that it is real, and that it will pass. Do not be embarrassed, alarmed, or feel guilty about your feelings. Discuss your depression openly and candidly with your doctor. Cut down on your social activities during the days or weeks following the birth of your baby. Enlist friends and/or family to help you out during the early weeks after your return from the hospital. Get plenty of rest. It can also take some pressure off you if you prepare healthy, well–rounded meals in advance to store in the freezer or refrigerator for use as necessary.

What should I do if the depression persists?

Contact a professional for help. Depression which lasts for several weeks or more, will warrant a visit to the doctor. If your depression is severe, your obstetrician or family doctor can refer you to a specialist who deals with these problems.

SLEEPLESS NIGHTS WITH BABY

Getting adequate rest and sleep when your newborn arrives, or when you have small children at home, is sometimes a bit more of a challenge when there's nobody there at 3:00am to help you. Being flexible, getting to sleep earlier at night, and taking cat naps when your child takes a nap is one of the best ways to fit extra rest into your hectic schedule.

Yes, you will sleep again!

Sometimes it's hard for a new mother to imagine that she will ever sleep again. Night after night of walking the floor, along with the other responsibilities of caring for baby, make sleep seem so inviting — and yet so elusive. This sleep deprivation may be one of your more difficult challenges. It may be a long haul, but rest assured, your baby will eventually adjust and you will once again be able to sleep through the night.

In the meantime, adjusting to your newborn's schedule may seem impossible. At times, it may even seem that you will go crazy from sleep deprivation. Unfortunately, our daily responsibilities don't stop just because we now have a new, demanding baby whose come to live with us!

> *"Paitence is the ability to idle your motor*
> *when you feel like stripping your gears."*
> Barbara Johnson
> *Where Does A Mother Go To Resign?*
> *(Bethany House)*

Baby's sleeping patterns.

For some babies, sleeping through the night occurs early on. For others it can take a lot longer. Most babies average approximately 16-18 hours of sleep a day, spread out in approximately five sleep cycles.

Within a few days of birth, many babies sleep for longer periods at night than during the day. By about two months, nearly half stay asleep for at least 5 hours during the night. And by the end of the first year, most infants will adjust to one long period of sleep at night with a morning and afternoon nap. However, every baby is different.

Until your infant adjusts to her big, new world, love, acceptance and cat naps will help you over the rough spots. Be patient. You will get through this.

If you find that acceptance is elusive and you become cranky, edgy, or angry — rest assured, these emotions are normal. I haven't met a mother yet who didn't lose her cool at some point in the early days. It's a natural part of the adjustment process.

Helping your infant to separate day from night.

Since your new baby will not be on your schedule in the beginning, it's best to adapt to your baby's sleep cycles. Years ago, mothers were taught to put their new babies on a strict schedule. But we have since learned that they are too young to be taught when to sleep. However, there are things you can do to help her separate night from day and adjust to a regular pattern of sleep:

- **Avoid overstimulation, play and entertainment at night.** Schedule day as "awake time" and night as "sleep time".
- **Put your baby in bed for sleep time.** Avoid allowing her to fall asleep in your arms, in a stroller or carrier. Condition her to understand that the bed is where she sleeps at night.
- **Adjust the lights.** Keep lights low or off at night. This will help baby to associate darkness with sleep time at night.
- **Adjust the room temperature.** Make sure the room is warm. If she gets chilly, she is likely to wake.
- **If she cries in the night go to her immediately.** While you attend to her needs, don't make a fuss and don't play or talk. Concentrate on gentle pats or cuddles instead.
- **Wrap her securely.** Wrapping your baby snugly in a blanket will help her to feel secure.
- **Make a ritual out of bedtime.** By bathing and changing her into nightclothes at the same time each evening, you will condition her to associate this ritual with sleep time. Regular feeding times should also be a part of this ritual.
- **Ordinary sound and activities will not disturb your newborn.** If you start off by tiptoeing about, talking in whispers, and taking the phone off the hook while she sleeps, there will come a time when your baby expects this silence. If you condition her from the beginning to sleep through normal sounds and activities, she will not be bothered by them later on.

What am I doing wrong? — Why can't I calm my baby down?

If your baby cries all the time for no apparent reason, he may have colic — and the fact is, you're probably not doing anything wrong. You are not responsible for your baby's crying. Crying is the only way your baby has to exert control over his environment, to make things happen, and to communicate. Although little is known conclusively about the cause of colic, the latest research indicates that colic has to do with your baby's development, and has nothing to do with you.

One of the best things you can do when your baby is screaming is to remain calm and rational — though that's not always easy. Nonetheless, it's important for you to try your best. Keep in mind that while you are not responsible for your baby's crying, he will pick up on your negative energies. Remaining calm may help him to calm down too. It may help you relax if you close your eyes and breathe deeply. And remember, at one time or another, every new mother feels inadequate to meet her baby's needs.

IDENTIFYING COLIC

Your baby may have colic if he does not just cry, but screams and draws his legs up to his belly. And while he may settle down for a minute or two, the screaming, shaking, and sobbing soon starts again. He may even drop off to sleep for a short period of time, but then wakes up screaming within a half an hour or so. These bouts of crying go on for as long as three to four hours, but then it is over and done with for the rest of the day (or night). This pattern repeats itself everyday about the same time.

Talk to your doctor about your concerns. He or she will examine your baby to make sure that there is no physical reason, such as pain or indigestion causing his to be distressed.

Frustration toward your colicky baby.

When I was a new mother, I thought I needed to be perfect, loving and patient at all times. After all, what kind of mother gets frustrated or angry at her new baby for crying? Well, I've learned a lot since then, and let me assure you, most mothers experience these feelings at least some of the time.

When your baby won't stop crying, when you've been up for several nights on end, and when nothing you do seems to calm him down, it can be utterly and painfully frustrating — particularly when no one is there to take the baby off your hands even for a little while.

You may feel helpless, or even desperate. You may even feel like lashing out. These moments can be very scary. Many mothers have uttered the words "I feel like throwing him out the window!" While having these thoughts is normal, *acting upon them is not*. You must do everything in your power to remain calm and keep your wits about you.

If you feel that you are going to lose control, or harm your child, seek help immediately. It is never appropriate or safe to shake, strike, or throw your child. If your fleeting thoughts become greater urges, go immediately to a neighbor's house and ask them to hold your child until you can pull yourself together. Or put your child down safely in another room and close the door. Then call your pediatrician or personal physician, a family member, therapist, or friend and tell them you are in trouble. Ask someone to come over right away.

If you can't find anybody who can come over, immediately call your local child–abuse hotline, found in the yellow pages under "Crisis Intervention Services", "Human Services Organizations", or "Parents Guidance Instruction". Call Parents Anonymous (909) 621–6184. Or call the Boys Town Child Abuse Hotline at (800) 448–3000. They offer a free, 24 hour hotline services to parents and children. You can speak to a highly trained counselor to discuss problems including abusive relationships; parent/child conflicts; depression; and frustration.

In any case, if you feel like you are losing control, it is important to call somebody — anybody — to help defuse the situation. Don't just sit there, and don't act on your impulse to *make* your child shut up.

Finally, if you continue to feel angry, hostile or resentful toward your child, seek help from a trained professional who can help you to deal with these feelings. Stuffing your feelings will put you at higher risk of eventually acting them out toward your child in an inappropriate manner. This will also diminish your opportunities to bond with your child. Furthermore, your angry or resentful feelings will cause you to feel badly about yourself, which in turn hurts your self–esteem.

Ideas to help you soothe your colicky baby.

Unfortunately, there is no sure cure for colic. There is no medication or herbal remedy that is guaranteed to solve the problem; and some may even worsen it. However, there are many things you can do to attempt to soothe her. The following may or may not help, but they are all worth a try.

- **Try to figure out the cause.** Is your baby hungry (perhaps undernourished), tired, or wet? Perhaps she's too hot or too cold. It may even be that she's bored or she's been in the same position for too long. Run through the possibilities to see if you can find the cause.
- **Respond to your baby.** Studies indicate that babies whose mothers respond quickly to them in infancy, tend to cry less as toddlers. Furthermore, if you can calm your baby before the crying intensifies, she will be more likely to settle down. Once her crying gets out of hand, it may be harder for you to figure out what started it in the first place.

  It is important for your baby to learn to trust that you are there for her. Meeting your baby's needs (even when it appears your attempts to comfort her do not soothe her) is the early foundation upon which your relationship is built. She needs to know that she matters; that she's important; and that you care.

  Don't worry about spoiling your young baby, at least during the first six (and some say twelve) months or so. Young babies cannot be spoiled. Your baby needs your consistent and prompt attention. As a result of your efforts, your child will be more likely to be trusting, confident and secure, and less likely to be overly demanding or dependent as she grows. Your tiny infant needs as much love and attention as she can get.
- **Rock your baby** in a rocking chair, cradle, or carriage. Rhythmic motions are very soothing for many babies. Many babies also respond to the motion of a baby swing, but you should not

put her into one before she is at least six weeks old. Rocking her up and down on your chest may also calm her, while rocking her side to side may stimulate her. *A word of caution:* be sure that you don't shake or rock your baby too hard, as it can cause serious — and sometimes fatal — injuries to your child.

- **Walk with your baby** in your arms, in a sling, a carrier, or a stroller. Simple enough, but it often works. In fact, studies show that babies who are carried for at least three hours per day cry less than those who are carried less often.
- **Take your baby for a ride in the car**. The motion of the car can be very soothing for a baby.
- **Swaddle your baby**. Newborns, especially, like to be wrapped snugly in a blanket. Ask the nurse to show you how to "wrap" your baby before you leave the hospital.
- **Hum and sing to your baby.** Your baby will likely respond to the sound of your voice — even if you can't carry a tune. Like adults, babies respond to different types of music. Find out what kind of music is soothing to your child.
- **Introduce your baby to a special "womb" song** before her birth. Your baby hears and responds to music while she is in your womb and will remember it after she is born. Studies indicate that a song sung, or played to a baby before birth, is calming to a baby after its birth.
- **Massage or stroke your baby.** Gently, but firmly rub her back, stomach, legs, or arms. Most babies are soothed by massage; however, some are not.
- **Pat your baby's back.** Lie her down on your chest, or hold her upright, and firmly pat her back (careful not to pat too hard.)
- **Give your baby a warm bath** — but only if she likes baths. Note that most newborns dislike being naked. If she cries after you take her clothes off, cover her with a towel or blanket before putting her in the tub. You may also notice that the sound of the running bathwater is soothing to your baby.
- **Rhythmic sounds are very calming to many babies.** It may seem strange, but the sound of a dishwasher, vacuum cleaner, or washing machine can be very soothing. A tape recording of nature sounds (wind, waves, rain, etc.) are also good bets. You can pick up "nature sounds" at nearly any music store.

Some ideas to help you cope with your crying baby:

- **Establish a routine.** For many babies, routines are helpful to reduce crying. Although you want to remain flexible, as your baby grows, by establishing a consistent routine, she can learn to anticipate her activities. This is comforting to infants, and may help eliminate unnecessary stress for both you and your infant.
- **Cut down on visitors or unnecessary stimulation.** If your baby is colicky, it may be a good idea to limit visitors and stimulating activities — particularly in the late afternoon and early evenings. Most babies tend to get fussy or downright agitated around the same time each day, and very often they let loose at the end of the day or in the early evenings.

  Some experts feel that babies tend to cry toward the end of the day or in early evenings because they are releasing the cumulative stresses and stimulations experienced during the day. If your baby has colic, try to keep her activities calm and as stress–free as possible.
- **Take a time out**. If nothing you do seems to help calm your baby, it may be helpful for you to take a time out. If you allow your baby to cry for 15 minutes in her crib, it will not harm her. Go to her after you have given yourself a little time to regroup.

  If the problem persists over a period of time, you can also purchase a pair of ear plugs to diminish the loud screams. Earplugs won't block out the crying altogether, nor would you want them to, but it will make the noise more bearable for you.

Enlist family and friends to stay over after your baby arrives.

If you have family or friends who can help you during the early days or weeks, by all means, accept their help. And if they don't offer, go ahead and ask. Perhaps you can even schedule your family and/or friends to each spend a day and night with you to help with the baby, the house, or the cooking, and enable you to get some much needed rest. This will be particularly helpful if you have had a caesarian.

Obviously you will not want to impose upon anyone. But chances are your loved ones will be happy to help you out for a day every so often. They may even expect you to allow them to help you. Use the time they liberate to really pamper yourself as you adjust to the huge changes in lifestyle demanded by a new baby. Not only will you feel better, but you'll likely feel closer to all of the loving hearts and hands around you. Your baby will appreciate them too, and will develop a natural trust for people around her.

It is also important not to worry if your house is not impeccably cleaned, that you can't seem to get out of your pajamas, or that you are too tired to do any cooking right after your baby's birth. It is natural that you will be drained. Taking care of a newborn is your main concern, so don't try to be superwoman. Choose to rest over being a perfect homemaker.

THE "FAMILY BED"

There are many advantages to sharing the family bed. Though sleeping with you will not stop your baby from waking up several times in the night, and it will not save you from night feedings, having him close to you will make feedings and diaper changing easier than if you have to get up and go to him.

Put a basket of diapers and diaper wipes next to your bed. If you are formula feeding your infant, a bottle prepared just before bed will not spoil overnight on the nightstand, and will be ready and on hand when your baby's hunger wakens him.

Sleeping together will encourage closer bonding. He will feel most safe, secure and comfortable being next to you. And being close to you will help him to get back to sleep more easily and quickly after he awakens for feedings. Furthermore, babies who sleep in the family bed tend to wake much less than other babies as they get older.

If you do decide to have your baby sleep in your bed with you, rest assured that it is highly unlikely that you will physically harm him for two very significant reasons. The first is that your natural instincts will keep you from rolling over onto your baby. The second reason is that your baby would surely wake up and cry if you were to accidentally begin to hurt him.

The downside to the family bed.

The downside to having your infant sleep in your bed is that when it's time to make the transition from mommy's bed to a bed of his own — your attempts may cause a miserable fight. He will likely throw a fit the first several times you put him into his own crib or bed. Children get very comfortable with their sleeping arrangements, and may not make the transition well.

CHILD CARE

If you plan to return to work, or if you must return to work as an economic necessity, then child care will be an important issue for you. You will want to devote enough time and attention to looking into day care as soon as possible to make sure that your child receives the best care possible.

Family can be the best answer to the child care dilemma.

If you have family who can offer child care to you, then you are among the fortunate. Having a family member care for your child generally provides many advantages that outside help may not be able to offer. Among other things, a family member is certainly a better economical value than hiring someone who is unrelated to you. More important is the fact that a family member is more likely to love your child. You know your family members' values, morals, and temperament much better than those of a stranger.

If you do not have a family member able or willing to care for your infant, you may discover that the combination of reliable, affordable, convenient, and loving child care, especially for a newborn, may prove to be difficult to find; but you can find it.

Child or day care centers.

When looking for suitable child care, it is a good idea to visit several child or day care centers so that you can determine if the setting, fees, hours, care giver's personality, etc. are acceptable to you and appropriate for your baby.

If you are planning to return to work soon after your baby's birth, it may be a good idea to begin looking for an appropriate day care center or provider prior to your baby's arrival so that you are not overwhelmed with this task once your baby is here. However, you still might want to bring your baby back after his birth to see how the care giver and staff reacts to and handles him before making your final choice between several options.

What to look for in a child care setting:

When looking for appropriate child care, consider the following:

- Is the day care facility licensed?
- What is the ratio of child care worker to child?
- What are the qualifications of the individual staff members?
- Is the environment set up for newborn babies, infants or toddlers?
- What are the age ranges of the children who are left in the care givers home or center?
- Will the care givers take an active role with your baby during the day or will they leave him in a crib?
- Are the meals provided for your older child? Are they hot meals?
- Is the facility or home clean? (Although cleanliness is very important, you should be wary of a center or home which is spotless or sterile. After all, the kids should be having a good time playing and one can't play in a sterile environment).
- Are there guards on windows above the ground level?
- Are there adequate, functioning fire alarms, smoke detectors, and fire extinguishes?
- Are there alternative exits for emergencies?
- Is the facility child–proofed?
- What are the hours, and what is the proximity to your home or office?

Trust your instincts. If you do not feel good about a situation, then look for another.

Alison, the single mother of a three year old has done just that. She moved on from several day care centers due to unacceptable conditions in each of them. "I've been very disappointed in day care."Alison exclaimed. "As a society, we pay a lot of lip service to what our children need, but we don't have adequate day care to back it up. Day care workers are grossly underpaid — which affects the level of performance."

If you don't find what you're looking for at the first — or third center — move on until you find an appropriate setting for your child. Don't settle for less.

Once you decide on a particular child care setting, you may want to make several surprise visits to see what is going on when they are not expecting you. It's also a good idea to have a back–up child care provider just in case your regular care giver becomes sick, goes on vacation, etc.

Where can I find child care in my area?

Ask friends, family and other parents for referrals. If you belong to a single mothers support group, this will likely be an excellent source for referrals. Many churches and synagogues sponsor child care programs — call and ask. Look in your local phone book under "Child Care Center" and "Child Care Consulting and Information Services".

You may want to consider taking out an ad in your local paper for a person in your area to watch your child(ren) in your home or theirs. An older person who has raised children of her own, and perhaps grandchildren, is also an excellent bet. You can ask another mother who is a stay–at–home mom if she's interested in taking on your child to earn some extra cash. Or if she has live–in help, maybe your child can stay there too.

In–home care givers.

If you can afford it, you can hire a nanny, au pair, babysitter, or housekeeper to care for your child in your home. However, this option is generally more expensive than day care centers.

Depending upon the area in which you live — and the care giver's qualifications — salaries for live–in help will range from approximately $500 – $2,400 per month (plus room and board). Care givers who do not live–in are paid in the range of $5.00 – $12.00 per hour. Some professional care givers will require insurance benefits, paid vacations and holidays.

If you hire someone to care for your child in your home, you will be required to withhold taxes (Social Security, state unemployment, and other taxes depending upon your state's requirements). And you will be required to report quarterly wages to the state. Some states require that in–home care givers be licensed. You can check with the human services agency in your state to determine the rules governing in–home care givers.

In–home care givers can live in or out, and can provide full or part–time care, depending upon your needs. In–home child care (particularly live–in help) offers many benefits — especially for working mothers. You will have more flexibility if you work late, and can more readily make plans to go out for an occasional date or get–together with friends. And you won't have to worry about driving to drop–off and pick–up your child at a day care facility.

If you hire someone who cleans your house and cooks in addition to providing child care, it will take a big load off of you. You will have more time to spend with your child. If you decide to hire live–in help, you can take out an ad in your local newspaper, or pay an agency fee to locate candidates.

When hiring domestic help, agencies are a good way to find prospective, qualified individuals. They will usually check references, criminal and driving records, and very often bond the individuals whom they refer to you (bonding is a duty or obligation imposed by a written contract).

Generally, an agency will require a fee of at least one month's salary if not more to place an applicant in your home. This route can be costly, but an agency will generally guarantee the placement for a specified period of time so that in the event a placement does not work out, they will refer someone else to you.

If you decide to find someone on your own, make sure you have an in–depth interview and check references carefully. Once you hire someone, spend time with her before you leave her alone with your child. Spending time with the care giver will give you a better idea of the type of person she is. Once you are ready to let her take over, you can drop by for unexpected visits or have family and friends drop by to check on things.

Child care tax credits.

Presently, the monthly child care allowance is $200. Thus, $200 of your monthly salary is non–taxable. Be sure to ask your accountant or employer how you can arrange to take advantage of this tax credit.

In case of emergency...

Make sure your care giver knows how to perform emergency cardiopulmonary resuscitation (CPR). If she has not been certified in CPR, there are many hospitals, schools, local parks and recreation, and other agencies which provide certified classes in emergency techniques. It would be a good idea to enroll her so that you have the added assurance that she knows how to handle an emergency. A CPR class is recommended for all new mothers as well.

Be sure to leave emergency telephone numbers for your care giver when you are away. Place the number of your doctor, hospital, work, family, friends, neighbors, etc., permanently next to the telephone where they can be easily found in an emergency.

You should also sign an authorization consent for the treatment of your child. Every child care worker or day care center should have this letter on file. This letter gives your care giver authorization to approve of emergency medical treatment for your child in your absence. Ask your doctor for a form letter, check with a stationery store, or write your own authorization letter indicating your doctors name, local hospital, and your caretaker's name.

ORGANIZING YOUR TIME

Effective time management.

Juggling the daily needs of children, career, a home, hobbies, and a social life can be very stressful. This "time crunch" can be a difficult, if not a painful hurdle to get over, particularly when you're single.

When a partner is not in the picture to help you with the daily responsibilities of your day–to–day life, it may seem nearly impossible to cope with this problem. However, you can find ways to make effective time management work for you.

Overcoming the time crunch, both emotionally and practically speaking, may seem a difficult, if not impossible task. After all, how do you stretch a limited amount of hours in a day to accommodate everything that needs to be done? I wish there was an easy answer.

Obviously you will have to do the best you can to accommodate your working schedule, chores, personal needs, and the needs of your child — and to deal with your feelings about all these pressures. Here are a few suggestions:

First things first – the "Master List".

The Master List is a list of things you need to do. It will be helpful if you get into the habit of carrying a small pad or spiral notepad with you wherever you go. This way you can write down anything and everything you need to accomplish as soon as you think of it. As you add to your list, you will want to break your items down in order of priority.

Your "A" list will consist of urgent gotta–get–it–done–yester-day things to do. Your "B" list will consist of important — but can wait–until–tomorrow — things to do; and your "C" list will contain necessary–but–can–wait–till–you–have–time items.

Each day, choose a few items from your "A" list to accomplish. Cross off your tasks as you accomplish them. It will give you a sense of completion. Look at your "A" list on a daily basis to update and move items up from your "B" and "C" list as appropriate. This will keep your list current.

Your list(s) will help you to remember things, prioritize and keep track of goals, and to accomplish tasks. Once you get into the habit of keeping a list and going over it, you will find the time spent reviewing your lists is well worth the accomplishments you make.

Month–at–a–glance.

Another helpful way to organize and prioritize, is to use a large month–at–a–glance calendar to write out your responsibilities and activities. Keep your calendar in a space where you can see it on a daily basis. This visual aid will help you keep track of chores, appointments and activities.

Recorded reminders.

If you can afford a hand–held recorder, carry it in your purse. Whenever you think of something to do, tape record it. Play it back while you're getting ready for work, while in the car, on your lunch break, or any other available time. Erase tasks as you accomplish them, or after you've written them on your Master List.

Accomplish multi–tasks.

Learn to do several things at once. Do your laundry while you cook, while the bath runs, while talking on loud speaker to a friend. Yes you can do it! Find ways to accomplish multi–tasks, instead of doing all things one at a time. Of course, many things need to have your full time and attention, and must be done one thing at a time. But many things can be done simultaneously. It can be fun to experiment with creative multi–tasks.

Learning to organize your time and accomplish multi–tasks will go a long way toward helping you to get things done faster and easier. And it will give you a sense of mastery. It will also provide you with more free time (of what there is) to spend with your child. Practice, practice, practice, and you will excel in the area of time management.

Make a file system and get organized.

Buy a cardboard box, or small file cabinet (you can purchase a second–hand cabinet at a used office furniture store), and folders. Make folders for bank statements, bills, income tax materials, insurance documents, personal data such as birth certificates and social security cards, etc. This will help keep you more organized, and you'll be able to find things when you need them.

Finish what you start.

Leaving tasks and projects half finished generally adds stress to our already hectic lives. When you start a task or project, see it through to completion. This will help to keep you on track. It will also make an impression on your child and influence his habits as he gets older.

Maximize your time.

Use occasional lunch hours to go to the dry cleaners, post office, drug store, etc. On your drive to work, leave a few minutes early to run simple errands. Eliminating the need to do these things on weekends will free up some of your time so you can spend it relaxing and having fun with your child.

QUALITY TIME WITH YOUR CHILD

"Quality time" has become a popular term in recent years, which seems to more accurately translate to mean: "I don't have enough time to spend with my child, so I make sure the time we do have together is of a high quality".

So what is quality time?

Quality time is time spent with your child that is dedicated to positive, child–oriented, age–appropriate, interactive play activities, or discussions, or togetherness. During this time you may choose to read to your child, play a board game, exercise, do sports, cuddle and talk, cook together, or even make a game of doing chores together.

This is your special time together that will hopefully enrich your child's life and leave a fond and meaningful impression on him. However, you don't have to drop everything at *all* times in order to spend quality time with your child.

You give your child quality time every time you feed, bathe, or change his diaper if you do these activities with patience, love, and good humor. You give him quality time even when you talk to him as you do your chores or cook dinner. Quality time is *not* time spent in front of the television, arguing, ignoring, or talking down to a child.

Quality time does not necessarily replace "quantity time". It is simply a way of condensing a limited amount of time into a positive experience. It is a time to share the best of you with your child.

Every moment does not need to be filled with activities or stimulation. Your child will be happy just to be with you. Your child should be able to count on this time together with you on a daily basis. And consistency in maintaining this ritual is vital.

Is quality time just a cop–out for those who choose not to take time to raise their children?

Many social critics believe that quality time is a convenient excuse for parents who choose not to spend much time raising their children themselves. It is interesting to note however, that many of those who do the criticizing appear to have the luxury of spending more time with their children due to flexible careers or two–parent families.

Unfortunately, many of us do not have those options. Quality time is not a cop–out, it is a necessity for many of us who must work in order to support our families, particularly when Dad is not in the picture.

For others, a career is a choice. Many women want to be mothers but also opt for a career. In these circumstances spending quality time with our children becomes a way of life. Whether you work by choice or necessity, you will need to work hard at finding available time to spend quality time with your child.

I feel guilty being away from my child — but I have to work.

Welcome to the club! Many mothers (even married ones) feel guilty about being away from their child. For working mothers in particular, guilt is a common emotion. When your child exhibits distress over your absence, it makes the situation even more difficult to deal with.

It can be very painful to deal with the guilt of being away from your child. But the reality is, the time you have left over is all the time you've got. Feeling guilty is not going to change your situation. You probably can't quit your job, so you must strive to make the best out the situation.

Adopting a positive attitude and being creative wherever possible, will go a long way toward strengthening your spirits. Nonetheless, even when you do find creative solutions which you feel pretty good about, a limited time schedule may still be very stressful on you and your child.

Here are some suggestions on ways to minimize the guilt and the problem:

- During the work week, set aside a portion of each day or night, to dedicate yourself 110% to your child whenever possible. Whether you can spare thirty minutes or four hours, your child needs this time with you.
- Having family time at dinner time seems basic enough, but with busy schedules, many single moms don't make this a priority. Turn off the T.V. and remove other distractions. Take this time to create family time with your child.
- Wake up (even fifteen minutes) earlier than necessary to begin your day. Take your baby for a walk in the stroller down the street, tumble on the floor together, enchant her with a favorite toy. With your older child, go outside and play catch; dance to music together; jog up the street together; or sit and chat. Early morning is a great time to connect with your child. It sets the tone for the day for both of you. This early morning time together is a good time to talk about your plans for the day, or simply do silly stuff together.
- Work on communication with your child. Active listening, sharing and caring is important to forging a closer relationship built on trust and respect.
- Involve your baby in your routines. Take her with you in the bathroom when you get ready for work; or into the bedroom when you change your clothes after work. Let her play with the grocery bags (non–plastic ones) while you put the food away, or play with child–safe kitchen utensils while you do the dishes.
- Dedicate as much time as possible on weekends to your child. While you will need some time alone for yourself, your child needs to know that she is a priority for you. Make weekends, holidays and vacations special times.

- Introduce your child to your own hobbies and interests whenever possible, or adopt your child's interests and hobbies. There are many hobbies even the youngest child can participate in. Gardening, cooking, dancing, reading, computer activities, etc. There are many things we can do with our kids, while we stimulate our own brains.
- If you are on a tight budget, find creative, free, or inexpensive ways to have fun. Your child needs you more than she needs any high ticket items, trips or excursions.
- If you cannot be there on any given day or night (perhaps you have a class or must work late), when your child is old enough to understand, let her know in advance that you'll be home late. If you can, take her to work with you for a day every now and then.
- Call your child from your workplace to tell her you love her.
- Send her special "love letters" by mail.
- Leave a note in her backpack (even a small child going off to day care will be delighted by a picture note from you.) You can ask your child care provider to share it with her.
- Make chores a fun time with your child. Cleaning house, laundry, cooking, washing the car (water fight) — anything you can think of can be turned into a game with a little bit of creativity. Play "I Spy" to clean up; have your little "master chef" help prepare the meal; have a tooth brushing contest — be creative.
- Let go of the need to have a spotless house in favor of spending more time with your child. Your child cares more about your attention than whether the furniture is dusted. While you don't want to live in chaos or filth, (nor is it good to teach your child that such living conditions are okay), there is a balance. Keep your expectations of your perfectly clean house in perspective.
- Give lots of cuddles and hugs. Invite your child into bed on Saturday mornings to snuggle, play or talk.
- Seek counseling if your older child displays anger or resentment over your not being there enough for her.
- Be creative with time management. Learn to incorporate activities. For example, take a bath with your baby; read a book

you're interested in aloud to your child (of course it should be child–appropriate); or have your older child help you clip grocery coupons.

- Be willing to forego personal plans or events in favor of spending time with your child. Giving up a portion of your freedom is one of the sacrifices that you have to make if you want to raise a happy child. The pay–off is really worth it over the long–term for both you and your child.

- The first time your baby cries as you close the door behind you (and you've got to get to work) — when that feeling of guilt rushes through the core of your being — take a deep breath, and trust that the love and nurturing you give your child through all the years of her life will help her to be all right.

> " *We make a living by what we get –*
> *but we make a life by what we give.* "

"Supermom"

In my own situation, I do not arrive home from work each night until nearly 6:30pm. Taylor needs to be in bed by 8:30pm in order to get enough sleep to be alert in school. The math is pretty clear here.

During the week, in the evenings I have two hours to spend quality time with Taylor. In this time, I need to go over his homework with him, read school bulletins, eat dinner, talk about the day (what he did at school, etc.), read or play a game with him, brush teeth (I've arranged to have his sitter bathe him before I get home), and finally say prayers before he hops into bed.

Two hours never seems to be enough time for these activities. Often I feel great pressure to cram it all into such a small time frame. Add to the mix the fact that I have a baby who also wants my attention, the phone may ring, and other distractions may occur — and you get the picture of a very hectic evening. Yet I attempt to faithfully follow this routine every week day — even on those days when I'm tired from a long day at the office and need a break.

Sometimes being "supermom" is an uphill climb and it's all I can do to keep my wits about me. I sometimes feel badly because I feel my children need more of me. And I feel sad when I miss big events in their young lives — such as Taylor's first steps — and finding out a day later that Jace's first teeth came in. But I do the best I can to accept my circumstance. I compensate where I can, and use quality time for all it's worth. Adopting a positive attitude is also important. Employing effective time management has also been essential in helping me to cope with the situation.

EXERCISE AND YOUR YOUNG CHILDREN

Developing habits that last.

Your young child or children will benefit from engaging in, and watching you enjoy and participate in active exercise. Your example and encouragement will help them to form their own habits and opinions about good health. They will be far more likely to develop good habits concerning exercise and fitness if they see you doing it.

In addition to setting a good example for your child, exercise is also a terrific way to spend fun, quality time together; so get your child involved in exercise activities with you. Children love to mimic us doing leg lifts, sit ups, jumping jacks, walking, running, etc.

Since most single mothers operate on a limited time schedule, where free time is at a premium, exercise is also a wonderful way for us to accomplish several things at once. When you exercise with your child, you simultaneously maintain and encourage better health, physical conditioning and emotional fitness.

At the same time, you spend positive, quality family time together, while improving coordination and teaching children good habits of health and body awareness. Because so many of our patterns and habits are developed when we are young, a child who is active as a youngster will be more likely to grow into a fit and active adult.

Engaging in sports with our kids is a great form of exercise. We commonly associate dads with teaching our kids to play baseball, football soccer, and basketball. Why not do it yourself? Most young children love playing sports and will enjoy them even more when mom's playing too. At the same time that we are teaching, praising and encouraging our kids to set goals, to be physically fit, to improve technique and coordination, we are also able having fun being active with them.

Times to remember.

The time you spend engaging in these activities with your child will likely be some of the most memorable times you spend together. Your kids will remember these occasions, even after they grow up, because this one–on–one time will be so special for them.

For you, the opportunity to share your child's sense of pride and accomplishment from learning to catch and throw a ball, make a basket, or make a touchdown will add up to many special memories. Because these activities require us to be physical, relaxed, and maybe even silly, there's not many better ways to be intimate, close, and to get "down and dirty" with our kids while meeting them at their level and having a great time.

KIDS AND EATING

The Eating habits of your growing child.

Nutritionally sound eating habits are important for your baby once she has been introduced to solid foods, for a good diet is essential for optimal health, development and growth. You will find that an early introduction to nutritional foods will make good eating habits easier to establish than if you try to change the tide after you have been lax in this area.

Just as your nutritional "habits" were formed in the early stages of your life, your child's habits will be formed early on, too. If you teach her to eat well now, she will be more likely to eat well throughout her life. Thus, it is very important to set the tone of her basic eating habits at a very early age.

When Taylor, my eldest son, was a baby, I decided I would keep sugar to a minimum. There is no grain sugar in the house. I only buy foods with little or no sugar in them. I stay away, as much as possible, from processed foods. And I watch the fat content in the foods I buy.

I do occasionally buy treats containing sugar, and even foods with no redeeming nutritional qualities whatsoever. However, I have found that Taylor, and my baby Jace, are (usually) just as happy with fruit juice sweetened products, fresh fruit, no sugar yogurt, popcorn, non–sugary cereal topped with fresh fruit, and natural juice popsicles (which I make) for afternoon snacks.

Like most kids, Taylor is greatly influenced by television commercials for those oh–so–exciting – got– to–have em' kid foods (Jace hasn't yet caught on to the allure of those commercials). To overcome this problem, we have learned to compromise. Once or twice a week, and on special occasions, Taylor gets to pick a "special treat". The rest of the time he eats lots of vegetables, fresh fruits, home-made soups (very easy to make!), grains, and pastas.

Instilling good eating habits.

When Taylor five years old, I began to play a sing–song game with him I called "Too much sugar!". We would put foods into a healthy "Good–for–you" group and a "Too much sugar" group (we also played this with "Too much fat", and "Too much processed" food groups). He loved the game and quickly began to understand the basic differences between healthy and not–so healthy foods.

Playing fun, animated games with your children to teach them about eating habits (and other subjects as well) is very impactful. If a child learns things in a colorful way, the lessons are more likely to be meaningful and remembered.

Moderation is best.

Healthy and fun treats are so easy to provide if we just give it a little thought. Still, I am convinced that if we deny our children any kind of "normal", unhealthy kid food, i.e., macaroni and cheese, hamburgers, french fries, cookies, potato chips, etc., they will rebel and find them at their friends' houses anyway. Moderation is best. While it is okay to give in to occasional treats, we should keep our eyes on our own — and our children's — healthy eating habits.

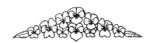

CHAPTER ELEVEN

YOUR CHILD'S DEVELOPMENT

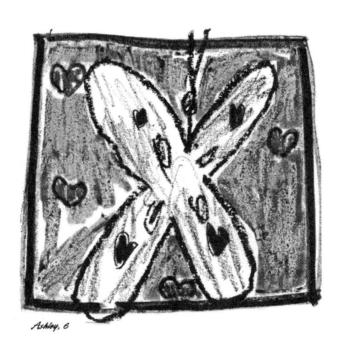

Ashley, 6

F I HAD MY CHILD TO RAISE ALL OVER AGAIN

If I had my child to raise all over again,
I'd finger paint more and point the finger less.
I'd do less correcting and more connecting.
I'd take my eyes off my watch, and watch with my eyes.
I would care to know less and know to care more.
I'd take more hikes and fly more kites.
I'd stop playing serious, and seriously play.
I'd run through more fields and gaze at more stars.
I'd do more hugging and less tugging.
I would be firm less often, and affirm much more.
I'd build self–esteem first, and the house later.
I'd teach less about the love of power,
and more about the power of love.

Diane Loomans

(From the book, Full Esteem Ahead: 100 ways to build Self– Esteem in Children
and Adults, written by Diane Loomans and her teenage daughter Julia, 1994.

HOW YOUR ATTITUDES AND BELIEFS AFFECT YOUR GROWING CHILD

Your child looks to you for cues and direction. He learns from
your example how to react to things in this world, and will model his
behavior after yours. To a great extent, your child's outlook on life
comes from your own beliefs and examples. Thus, it is particularly
important for you to look at the way you operate, and how you deal
with things.

A positive person has positive energy to share. This is a wonderful foundational outlook to provide for your child. In such an atmosphere it is much easier to teach him how to take responsibility
for himself. He will become a self–respecting, loving, emotionally
balanced, and caring individual if you possess and model these qualities in your everyday life.

Giving your child the greatest gift of all.

The best thing you can give to your child is the knowledge that he is loved and respected. It is your job to instill within him the belief that he is a worthy, important, and wonderful person. When your child possesses self–confidence and strong self–esteem, the challenges and problems that he will inevitably face in life will be far more manageable than if he has no strong foundation to support him through his difficulties.

A strong foundation is a necessity if he is to become a productive, self–sufficient and loving adult, and eventually a parent himself. We want our children to believe in themselves and to believe that their good thoughts and ideas can truly contribute to creating positive experiences.

What if I make mistakes?

As a parent, you will make mistakes (you can be sure of this.) At times, you will likely even use poor judgment. You may say things you wish you could take back, and you will probably act in ways that you regret. But fortunately, most children are remarkably resilient, loving and forgiving people. So don't give up.

None of us are perfect parents; but we can challenge ourselves to keep doing better. If you make a mistake, don't be afraid to say to your child "What I just did was not the best way I could have handled this situation. I'm sorry and I'm going to try again."

PARENTING CLASSES

*"Having children makes you no more a parent
than having a piano makes you a pianist."*
Michael Levine,
Lessons at the Halfway Point (Celestine Arts)

Child rearing is the most important task you will ever perform, yet it is one for which you will have the least preparation. Most of us learn how to be parents through on–the–job training, and by following the examples that our own parents set (which can be a good or not–so–good thing depending upon the skills of our parent(s).)

While some of you will take to parenting like a fish to water, others will not be as comfortable or intuitively prepared to be a mother. But no matter how prepared you may feel, the realities of bringing a baby home when you have never had such a huge responsibility can be an overwhelming experience. Not having a partner with whom you can share ideas, may also leave you feeling at a disadvantage.

All of your circumstances — including your financial condition, career, emotional well–being, temperament, and general character will also have an impact on your parenting experience. You will need to re–adjust your lifestyle and to re–think and re–learn certain ideas and attitudes about yourself, your life, and child–rearing.

Where's my manual!!!

Unfortunately, babies do not come with an owner's manual when we check out of the hospital. So whether we are married or single, we all need to learn to be good and better parents by utilizing the many resources we can find around us in order to create the best experience possible.

If you are feeling ill at ease with your abilities to be a good parent, and you feel the need to talk over your questions and concerns with someone, you may want to consider taking a parenting class or to seek help from other sources in your community.

Even the greatest athlete needs a coach.

If you think you are so together that you do not need instruction or help with your parenting skills, remember that even the greatest athlete needs a coach. Whatever it takes to do the best you can for your children, it is your responsibility to do so, even if it means letting go of your ego long enough to reach out to others for help.

The benefits of parenting classes.

Parenting classes offer great ideas — many of which you may not have previously considered. The focus of a parenting class is to help you improve your parenting techniques, and to teach you how to deal more effectively with the everyday, practical aspects of parenting.

You will learn valuable communication skills and techniques to improve your interactions with your child. You'll get help you with your temperament and may increase your ability to be patient with your child. You can learn wonderful, helpful tips; better understand your child and his needs; and share your feelings with other parents in the class.

Taking a parenting class demonstrates your love for your child.

Even if you have already had experience in raising a child or children, a parenting class may still be something to consider. Seeking new ideas, and sharing your experiences in a learning environment will help to improve your parenting skills. It's also a way to demonstrate to your child how very much you love him.

Taking a parenting class does not mean that you are an inadequate mother or a bad parent. Quite the contrary. Your decision to attend a class indicates your desire to be better at your job as a parent. It indicates that you care deeply enough about your child to improve yourself through education. And it shows that you desire to offer your child the very best of you.

Parenting classes are often offered by your hospital, local YMCA, private businesses, and other social service agencies.

TEACHING VALUES

Every family has expectations of behavior that are determined by principles and standards. These add up to values. Instilling values in your child will enable her to be a better person with a greater capacity for compassion, honesty, integrity, warmth and love. Some ways you can help to make your family's values clear are:

- **Communicate values openly.** Talk about why values such as honesty, responsibilities and self–reliance are important. Make it clear to your child why values will help her to make good decisions. Teach her how each decision builds upon a previous decision; and how a good decision makes the next decision easier. Let her know there are no short–cuts and nothing in life is free.

- **Recognize how your actions affect the development of your child's values.** Your child will mimic your behavior. For example, if you smoke, your child is more likely to smoke. Evaluate your own use of foul language, honesty, integrity, use of tobacco, alcohol, prescription medicines, illegal drugs, etc. Consider how your own attitudes and actions may be shaping your child's choice about such things.

- **Look for discrepancies between your words and your actions.** Even a very young child is capable of recognizing or sensing when a parent sends signals (by their actions) that it's alright to be dishonest or to shirk unpleasant responsibilities. Telling your child to say that you are not home when the phone rings, gives her the message that it's okay to tell even "white lies." Telling the gal at the theater counter that your child is still under age to get a free ticket, sends the message that it's okay to cheat.

- **Make sure your child understands your family values.** Don't assume that your child has absorbed your values. Discuss common values or situations at the dinner table or just before bed.

  With your younger child, talk about the need to control behavior (not hitting, throwing tantrums, etc.) Ask your older child of 5 or 6, questions such as: "What would you do if you found a wallet with money in it?" Let your child know that courtesy is important; taking turns is appropriate; and sharing is expected. Discuss all the "value" behaviors that are important to you.

DISCIPLINE

What is discipline?

The word *discipline* is derived from the Latin word meaning "to instruct" or "to teach." (Compare the word to *disciple*.) It does not mean to shame or humiliate. And for the purposes of this section, discipline is *not* intended to mean hitting or spanking.

Using corporal punishment is a personal choice. But it is one that I — along with many professionals — do not promote. Instead, discipline, as discussed herein, is intended to be utilized as a constructive method for discouraging undesirable behaviors — and encouraging desired behaviors within our children.

As a parent, you have an obligation to discipline your child in the way of family values by setting boundaries. Boundaries will help your child to develop self–control, character, respect for others' rights, orderliness and efficiency. Without boundaries, children are abandoned to their own immature impulses, and disharmony results and reflects in their relationships to people, places and things.

Experts tell us that children need to have boundaries in order to feel secure. Boundaries provide a dependable "container" within which the child can safely grow in his understanding and interaction with his world.

The firm but gentle embrace of reasonable boundaries let the child know that he is loved, cared for, and protected. By learning to recognize and respect your boundaries, your child will be more likely to inherit your values and will eventually express them in all of his other relationships.

Building the foundation of mutual respect early on will give you a leg up on creating a better relationship between you and your child. The later you start to instill good discipline (or boundaries), the more difficult it will be to accomplish — especially as your child grows older and begins to develop more independent thinking. So, begin at the beginning. And, most of all, love and appreciate your child through all of the difficult stages of his development.

The diversity of discipline.

Methods and philosophies of discipline have been hotly debated for centuries. Because the techniques of discipline are so varied and experts often disagree with each other, it's no wonder so many parents are quite confused when it comes to this issue. Common questions a parent might ask are: "What is the best form of discipline?"; "Why won't my child listen to me?"; and "When and how should I punish my child?"

Unfortunately, there are no pat answers to these questions. Ultimately, discipline is a very personal subject. And you will need to become well–informed in order to decide what approach is best for you and your child.

Keep in mind that to a great extent, your automatic approach will reflect what you experienced as a child. Your own parents may have been very effective disciplinarians — or you may have had cruel, ineffective role models. Awareness is particularly important in the latter case, in order that you not re–visit abusive discipline upon your child. The question to ask yourself is: "Will my approach offer my child the best opportunities for optimal growth and development? Or is it just my way of taking my upset out on my child — as my parents did with me?"

Some methods of discipline.

- **Traditional/Authoritarian.** This type of "no–nonsense" parenting style dominated our nation's history until post–World War II. It was brought to America with the European immigration of the late 1800s and early 1900s. In this style, the parent(s) are the ultimate authorities, making all of the important (and unimportant) decisions, while the children obey without question. There are clear cut distinctions and boundaries between the parent and child; the parents lead and the child follows. Child–development specialists suggest that this method is too harsh and produces too many repressed, neurotic children.

  Child development expert, John Bradshaw, points out that demanding unquestioning obedience to authority is *not* the kind of value we want to instill in our children, for this is counter–productive to a democracy.

- **Permissive.** This method, in its extreme form, is the exact opposite of the traditional/authoritarian style of parenting. This method was popular in the late 1940s, 1950s, and 1960s, and continues to be used by many parents today.

  The belief system of this style is that kids should be free from parental "control" and left to make up their own minds about (basically) everything. Parents who use this technique believe that the child will develop their natural talents and realize their greatest potential in life.

  However, most experts agree that this method does more

harm than good. Children raised in these environments tend to get into trouble at school, in their neighborhoods and with the law, because they never learn appropriate behaviors and important boundaries.

- **Alternating.** This method is not uncommon, and many parents make the unfortunate mistake of falling into this trap. In this method, a parent switches from traditional/authoritarian to permissive, and back again, often without rhyme or reason.

  The problem with this style is that children are left completely and utterly confused about the rules (or lack thereof), and never quite know where they stand. There is no set standard or predictable, reliable limit on their behavior.

  While no parent is ever 100% consistent in their parenting, nor are they expected to be, in this style of parenting, the inconsistency demonstrated to a child creates insecurity and undermines confidence.

- **Participatory**. In this style of parenting, the parent is firm, consistent, remains in charge, and provides clear–cut family leadership. But, the child is invited to contribute ideas and participate in the decision–making process.

  This style can be most effective, because while there are clearly defined rules, boundaries and methods of enforcement when rules are broken, the child is *heard,* and *listened* to.

Your child has a *need* to explore the world around him.

It is essential to your child's development that he be free to grow and learn by exploring the world around him. He needs to be able to use his imagination, experiment, and learn from his mistakes. It is your job as a good parent to encourage and nurture these qualities within him.

Your "role" as role model.

As we've already discussed in the section on "Teaching Values", it is vital that you model the very qualities you hope to instill within your child. In order for your child to learn honesty, integrity, patience, respect, responsibility, values, morals, manners and self–discipline, you must demonstrate these very qualities in your own daily affairs.

Your child will not take you very seriously if you expect these things from him but do not adhere to them yourself. It's also important to recognize that children readily see beneath surface appearances and won't be fooled by phony behavior.

Getting a head start.

Setting the tone for these lessons is critical in your child's younger years. Even your young baby is capable of responding to your cues and directions. And certainly by the time he is a year old, he is beginning to understand acceptable and appropriate behaviors. Of course he has limited self–control at this age, but nonetheless, he is very impressionable and teachable.

STRATEGIES TO SUCCESSFUL DISCIPLINE

A positive approach to successful discipline, is to avoid the need to punish your child. Some techniques to help you are:

- **Let your child know where he stands.** You should be consistent in your expectations of his behavior. If you keep changing the rules, he will become confused, resentful and even rebellious. He needs to be able to anticipate the rules.
- **Be a good listener.** Make sure your child feels comfortable bringing problems or questions to you. Listen closely to what your child says. Don't allow anger at what you've heard to end the discussion. If necessary, take a 5 minute break to calm down before continuing. Take note of what your child is *not* saying. If your child does not tell you about his problems, it may be an indicator that something is not right. Take the initiative to ask questions about what is going on.
- **Give your child explanations for rules.** Help him to understand why you have certain rules and allow him to ask questions about them. When discussing the rules (or answering his

questions) give him straight answers. Respect his intelligence. Your guidance will help him to understand and follow your instructions.

Telling your child "Because I said so" will not encourage the response you want. He will not learn anything useful from this statement and will likely resent you for saying it.

- **Teach limits.** After you explain the rules, make sure your child understands them and that he understands exactly what you expect of him. You may need to enforce these limits when he breaks them with logical consequences.

- **Be consistent in lavishing praise for appropriate, desired behaviors.** When you praise desired behavior (while it occurs — and after), it will help to eliminate the need for undesired behavior. If you are quicker to praise than to criticize, your child will learn to feel good about himself, and he will develop self–confidence and trust his own judgment.

For example, if Johnny tends to fight with the neighbor's child when they get together to play, instead of waiting for the fighting to begin, you would praise Johnny *while he is playing nicely*. With practice, you will find that you can anticipate a lot of your child's undesired behavior in advance of its occurrence, and take steps to head it off.

In this case, you might say: "Gosh Johnny, I just love the way you are playing with Alex. It is so nice to see you getting along so well. You are terrific!" You may want to hug him, smile, and show a genuine interest in his *desired* behavior.

It may take several times of trying this approach before the undesired behavior (fighting) stops. In the meantime, without yelling or making a big deal of the fighting, remove him from the scene, and in a very calm manner, simply say: "You must learn to play nicely with people." Do not allow your child to draw you into a debate. Just remove him from the activity while keeping your communication with him about the problem simple.

After you have done this several times, you will begin to see how the "carrot" of pleasing you is more rewarding for your child than the "stick" that comes when he displeases you. Remember, the more excited or angry you get, the worse the behavior often becomes.

- **Use distractions/substitutes.** You can avoid many battles with even your youngest child by offering something that is more appealing than what he's doing. For example, if your young baby is crying because you just took a sharp pencil out of his hands, replace it immediately with something safe and interesting. Or turn on some music and begin to dance around. If he likes music, he will forget the darned pencil in an instant. Try new approaches, be creative.

- **Child–proof your house or apartment.** If you reduce the potential for conflict by removing tempting or dangerous objects from reach, there is less likelihood for problems. And, you will not need to say "NO!" so often.

- **Limit access to certain activities and objects.** If you don't want paint all over the house, don't leave the paint can within reach! If an older child leaves a toy with small pieces around and your young baby may find them — remove them so that this conflict and potential hazard do not exist. If your very small baby is attracted to forks (like mine is) remove them from the table at a restaurant *before* he notices them.

- **Make a game out of discipline.** Enlist your child in participating in his tasks or chores by making it fun for him. If the task becomes more appealing to him, you may just avoid the need to remind or reprimand. For example, when putting toys away, have a race to see who can pick up the most, the fastest.

- **Repeat rules.** Your young child does not have the ability to remember things the first, second, or even third time around. He is learning so many new things on a daily basis, that you can't expect him to remember things the way an older child or adult would. Repeat rules and instructions often.

- **Criticize the behavior, not your child.** Experts recommend that we state our upset over a situation or behavior without turning it into criticism or an attack against the child. Try not to get into blaming your child: "I am so angry at *you*...because *you*..."; or name calling (such as "bad boy"). Instead convey the message that "I feel angry about this situation" Helping your child to understand that anger (within reason) is a normal, and healthy emotion, and showing him positive ways to express it, is important to his development.

- **When you are angry, express it in non–destructive, non–violent ways.** You are expected to get angry and you are entitled to express it. Just make sure that you do so in nondestructive, non–violent ways.

  Likewise, you will need to respect your child's right to feel anger and express it appropriately. Pounding clay, batting balls, pulling weeds, drawing pictures, journaling, etc., are all ways that you and your older child can ventilate.

- **Demonstrate desired behaviors.** Show your child — through your own example — what behaviors you expect from him. "Do as I say, not as I do" is not going to get your child to behave as you desire.

- **Tips on offering rewards for desired behaviors.** While it's nice to offer your child rewards for good behavior — and they often deserve them — they should not get into a "habit" of *expecting* them. Further, be careful not to give rewards for (or give–in to) undesired behavior. Your child will get the message that he gets extra attention for it.

- **Don't make such a big deal over the little things.** It's not possible to ignore all undesired behaviors and focus exclusively on positive behaviors. But it is possible to minimize our responses to the minor infractions of our rules. If you allow yourself to over–react to everything, you provide your child with a sure–fire way to push your buttons whenever he's seeking to "get" you.

- **Talk to your child in a respectful manner.** You can be very effective when you talk to your child in a calm and rational voice. This also conveys your respect for your child as a person. You do not have to yell to get your message across.

  Of course, you will yell sometimes. You're human. But if it is your primary mode of communication, you might want to take a look at its effectiveness and impact. If your child behaves but is emotionally scarred — what have you accomplished?

  You are a role model, and should act like one. Your behavior is key to developing your child's attitude and character. If you feel like you are going to lose control, it might be a good idea to take a break — even if only for a moment.

- **A cool down period.** Removing yourself from your child to cool down and think about what you are going to do about a particular problem might just help to diffuse the situation. Even when your child is a baby, you may need to go into another room to gather your wits about you.

  It is natural for you to feel like you will go nuts even with your small infant. After all, they are very demanding. Separating yourself from your child can help you to regain control over your emotions and feelings about what is going on, and to act in a more reasonable manner.

- **Say what you mean and mean what you say.** *Always, always,* say what you mean and mean what you say! Think about what you're going to say before you offer empty threats. If you make empty threats and don't follow through on them, your child won't take you seriously — and his behavior will reflect it. He will be inclined to "angle" to get you to change your mind (because he thinks he can).

Sometimes a more direct, firm approach to discipline is necessary.

Your child is going to act in ways that are not acceptable you. You will likely lose your patience many times over and find need to punish certain behaviors or actions. When your child's father is not in your lives to support you in those moments and to reinforce your authority, the subject becomes all the more important for you to deal with effectively.

Punishing your child.

After all other attempts have failed, punishment may be the only message that gets through to your child. In trying to figure out what punishment(s) your child responds to, it's advisable to be flexible in your approach, open to suggestions, and willing to discard methods that don't seem to work toward the achievement of your ultimate goal: the appropriate behavior of your child — achieved without injury to his self–esteem.

Here are some suggested approaches to punishment:

- **Time out.** If you are not getting the result you want with the more gentle approach of encouraging desired behavior, then you may want to try using a "time out". The accepted rule of thumb here is that you give your child one minute of time out for each year in age. You do not want to sit her in a corner facing the wall. But you do want to sit her down in a place where she will not be able to play with toys, watch T.V., etc. Time out can be an effective means of discipline, but you will not want to over use it.

  Here again, it doesn't help things if you scream or yell because that's not the kind of behavior you want to encourage. Instead you may want to calmly say something like: "You need to have a time out. Your behavior is not acceptable. Please go to your room and sit down on the chair for three minutes." Then let her know when her time is up.

  Again, no debates or prolonged conversations. In the beginning your child may cry as a means to manipulate you. Don't buy into it. You are in control here, not your child.

- **Taking away privileges.** Taking away a privilege is a very reasonable and effective approach in some situations. Depending upon the situation, you may take away a privilege for a short term or take it away indefinitely, but this "punishment" should fit the circumstances.

  For example, if your child will not eat her dinner, you may want to simply and casually say: "Fine, you don't have to eat your dinner, but you don't have to eat dessert either." If she continues to refuse to eat, take her plate away from the table. *Do not* give in later and give it back to her. (she will not starve if she does not eat one meal, I promise!)

  Another example might be to say: "If you can't play nicely with your brother, then you may not play at all." Children need to learn that there are consequences for their actions, and again they need to believe you mean what you say.

- **Be Consistent.** Applying these techniques is very effective if you are consistent. Consistency is important to our children and to their development. They need to be able to count on us, and to see that certain causes have certain effects.

A PARENT'S FRUSTRATION

As a parent, you can be guaranteed that you will experience frustration. Some feel it more than others, but life is full of frustration for everyone.

Your baby will cry, be demanding, and temperamental — all without as much as a thank you! Your toddler will break things, spill things, soil the shirt you just washed, throw temper tantrums, refuse to eat, and say "NO!" many times over.

As she gets older, your child will *really* give you a run for your money. She'll try to stretch boundaries and assert her independence. It's part of her job as a child to do these things — and yours to expect it. Expecting and accepting these things as part of the package will help you to reduce frustration.

Being aware of *what* triggers your frustration and *how* you react to it is important in keeping matters under control. While frustration is normal, acting it out in inappropriate ways is not.

A PARENT'S ANGER

I get really angry at my child, and I'm not sure I'm handling it very well.

All parents gets angry at their children. However, it's what we do about our anger, and how we express it on a continuing basis that makes the difference.

Expressing anger or displeasure in a rational and appropriate manner should be every parent's objective, for it releases tension and provides our children with a healthy demonstration of appropriate behavior.

However, you needn't worry about occasional, short–lived outbursts. You are human, and as such, you are allowed your share of frailties. As long as your outbursts are relatively few and far between, they should not leave lasting emotional scars on your child. However, if you fly off the handle on a regular basis with your child, or you act out in violence, these are serious signs that something is very wrong and needs to be addressed.

It is important for you to be aware of how you react to your child when you are angry. When moments of high anxiety or anger occur, it is necessary to remember that your long–term goal is to teach appropriate behavior.

If you deal with anger by screaming, yelling, hitting, slamming doors, or breaking dishes, what does this teach your child? What is your behavior telling her? Is this how you want to see her deal with her upsets?

When you find that you are angry at your child (and you will be — many times throughout her young life) there are a few good rules to remember:

Rule number one: Take a time out. Slowly breathe in and breathe out. Count to ten or even count to twenty before responding to something unacceptable. Call a friend. Splash some water on your face, and take a few deep breaths. Walk into another room for a moment to gather your wits about you before you tend to the problem.

Rule number two: Stay calm. A broken dish can be replaced. A stain in the carpet (hopefully) can be removed. These are tangible objects and only have the value we place upon them. Our child, however, is invaluable.

Rule number three: Remember your child is only a child and needs room to make mistakes. She needs to feel loved even when she's made an error.

Rule number four: Again, let your child know that her *behavior* is inappropriate, but do not tell her that *she* is bad. Explain to her what she did wrong, and why. Even a young child, while she may not understand your words, will understand your intention.

Rule number five: An accident is different from intentional disobedience or wrongdoings. If your child breaks a glass pitcher while trying to pour herself a drink, she already knows she made a mistake. If you get angry, she will learn guilt and fear. But if you gently tell her "Accidents happen — I'm sure glad you didn't hurt yourself", she will learn that *things* don't matter as much as your love for her and that it's okay to make mistakes. Don't make a big deal out of unimportant matters.

Rule number six: Find the bright side in every possible situation. Look for the silver–lining. Find a reason to laugh at yourself. Don't let anger take over your life. Life shouldn't be taken so seriously all the time!

Rule number seven: If you are unable to deal responsibly and reasonably when you are angry, get help!

A little story with a big moral:

A child of three, paints a beautiful paper butterfly for his mommy, whom he loves so much. "Oh" she says, "This is the *most* wonderful, beautiful butterfly I have ever seen! I will put it on the refrigerator where I will treasure it always. You are the best, most creative artist I've ever seen!" The child beams with pride. He's made his mommy so happy.

A few days later, with a big desire to make his mommy as happy as she was when he made her the paper butterfly, he decides to make an even better, bigger picture. With his crayons, he begins the greatest masterpiece of all! A picture *this big* on the wall.

He is so excited. In his tiny little mind, he thinks to himself: "This will make my mommy *sooooo* happy!" But when his mommy see's the picture; crayons of every color smeared across her newly painted wall, she doesn't think it's so beautiful.

The little boy's mommy gets so angry that she screams and yells — saying to her son: "You are a bad boy! How could you ruin my wall like that? I'm so angry at you. After you clean the wall, you will go to bed without supper!"

The moral: *Don't break the spirit of the child whose dreams you helped to create.*

ACCEPTING YOUR CHILD'S INDIVIDUALITY

As your child grows, there will be countless times when he will not do or be what you want him to do or to be. Undoubtedly, you will not always agree with his point of view, or the way he wants to dress and wear his hair. You can bet that there are going to be many areas of disagreement between you and your child, especially as he seeks to differentiate himself from you.

There will likely be a phase when peer pressure greatly affects your child. His desire to "fit in" and be a part of the group may sometimes conflict with your own ideas for him. When these situations arise, allowing your child to have a say in areas that are a matter of personal preference (i.e., hair, clothing, etc.) is important. You will want to encourage independent choice *without* denigrating his choice to be like everybody else.

Showing your child that you respect his independence and his ability to make certain decisions for himself will help to build his self–esteem and confidence. And giving him some lee–way in matters of personal expression will also go a long way toward enriching your relationship with him.

The process of "letting go".

As your child gets older, the process of "letting go" will be easier on you if you teach him (as a preschooler) how to make his own decisions and develop problem solving skills. It's tempting for busy parents to do things for young children (because it's easier or quicker). But with a little planning, you can use the learn–by–doing approach to teach your youngster to make appropriate decisions. This will help to ensure better decision making skills when he gets older and wants and *needs* more freedom to explore and experiment.

Let your child pick from a range of options that are acceptable to you. When the choice is made, make sure your child sticks with it — though some flexibility is reasonable.

While you will naturally set certain rules and expect certain behaviors, where matters of personal expression are concerned, it will serve you both better to allow him to pursue his own path (when it does not harm him or another) in the spirit of encouraging his independence.

When you consider the fact that you will say "no!" to your child thousands of times in his life for reasons of safety, health, education, and development, it is reasonable to say "yes" sometimes to the little things that don't matter so much — and to grant your child some independence and freedom of expression.

A compromise.

My rule of thumb is this: if the choice does not endanger anyone or contradict my basic principled beliefs, (i.e., honesty, integrity, compassion, etc.), I tend to say "yes" and allow the individual expression.

Sometimes, as leverage, I have my son, Taylor, "earn" the right to choose in a given situation. For example, if he gets himself ready for the school bus on time in the morning without prodding and constant reminders, I may let him choose the movie we will see over the weekend as an acknowledgment of his good deeds and diligent efforts.

A few years ago, my nephew's grades were slipping in school. So my sister made an agreement with him that if his grades rose over a given period of time to B's (which he was certainly capable of), then he could get his ear pierced. She didn't necessarily want him to have a pierced ear, but she knew how important it was to him. So instead of denying him the pierced ear, she looked at his desire to have one as an opportunity for both of them to get what they wanted. The incentive for him was so great that his grades rose within a matter of weeks and he now wears a stud in his earlobe.

Avoiding unnecessary battles.

You will likely notice that when you allow your child to have a say in certain matters, you will avoid many unnecessary battles, tears, and resentments. You will also see how using these situations as opportunities to encourage desired behaviors in your child will help to improve his level of responsibility, self–worth and respect for you. They will also teach *you* more about tolerance and acceptance.

FEARING FOR YOUR CHILD'S SAFETY

I am so afraid my child will get hurt — either physical or emotionally — it's a scary world out there!

As a mother, there will be countless times when you fear for your child. You may worry that she will be hurt by another, have an accident, be psychologically harmed by the lack of a father, among other things.

These feelings are normal and will serve to keep you on the

lookout for warning signs of danger and trouble. Hopefully, they will keep you tuned–in to your child — and keep you on your toes — always looking to improve the opportunities and resources you provide to your child.

Of course, as your child grows, it is necessary for you to talk about certain dangers. Telling a young child about the dangers of strangers, inappropriate touching, drugs, alcohol, and even crossing the street is diligent parenting. These are necessary, pro–active steps we must take as parents to better protect our kids. But *living* in fear and dramatizing the danger is very unhealthy for you and your child.

When you project perpetual fear to your child, you stifle her growth and teach her to live in fear. This will inhibit her creativity, expression, and exploration of the world around her.

Again, look at the messages concerning fear which you project — even to your young baby — by the things you do and say. Your attitude and projection will have a lot to do with the way she perceives her world.

I like to think of life and the world we live in as a series of miracles. To live in fear, and worse — to teach fear — diminishes the brilliance of those miracles of life. Be cautious, but do not live in fear.

IDENTIFYING POTENTIAL PROBLEMS IN YOUR CHILD

Identifying problems (or potential problems) in our children is important if we are to avoid allowing them to spiral out of control. By becoming aware that there may be odds against our children and ourselves as single–parents, we give ourselves a very important edge in making better overall decisions and overcoming the odds.

Knowledge is power, and forewarned is indeed forearmed. In attempting to understand what we are up against as single–parents, we can work on improving our parenting skills, attitudes, and resources. And we can then take action to find solutions which will help us avoid future problems with our kids.

Are there warning signs that my child may be in trouble? How do I identify the symptoms?

Oftentimes, your child will give you signals through his behavior that something is troubling him. Unfortunately, like adults, children do not understand many of their emotions and cannot articulate that they are in distress. They depend on your watchful eye and intervention. Some of the signs are clear and easy to detect. Others are more subtle. Emotional distress is no respecter of age. It can affect children as young as four or five as well as teens and adults.

If your child displays any of the following symptoms, it could be an indication that something is wrong. They can include:

- depression
- noncommunication
- moodiness
- overeating – or not eating
- difficulty staying focused in school; problems with ability to learn.
- complaints about physical symptoms (stomach aches, headaches, and dizziness)
- complaints about how "unfair" life is
- lying, stealing, cheating
- aggression, bullying, hostility, anger
- short temper
- withdrawal/isolating
- difficulty making friends
- exaggerated fear of people/places/things
- obsessive–compulsive behaviors
- frequent nightmares
- bed wetting
- feeling overly worried about things

If you suspect that your child is experiencing ongoing problems such as these, it is vital that you get professional help for him. When left untreated, these problems can lead to undesired behaviors, more serious forms of depression, and ultimately, bigger problems for you and your child down the road.

For a referral to a mental health professional in your area, you can call or write to the American Academy of Child and Adolescent Psychiatry, 3615 Wisconsin Avenue NW, Washington, DC 20016, (202) 966–7300.

Don't become overly frightened or paranoid either.

While it is important that you are aware and reasonably informed about potential problems, at the same time you *do not* want to become overly frightened or paranoid. As previously discussed, living in fear or insecurity is not healthy and doesn't promote happiness. Instead, you can allow yourself to become empowered by this information and learn from it.

You can begin by asking yourself how you can help your child avoid such difficulties. Take a look at what actions you can take to become a better role model, parent, teacher, provider, and what resources you can pull from to help you to achieve this goal.

Just as denying a potential problem doesn't make it go away, acknowledging it doesn't make it worse. It may just look that way at first. Furthermore, while single–parenting may invite potential problems, it does not mean that you are predetermining or accepting that you are headed for disaster or that you will have troubled kids.

To the contrary, by keeping an eye on potential problems, you will greatly improve your chances of avoiding future difficulties because you will be sensitive to the danger signs. If you catch the warning signals early, it is easier to remedy the problem with the help of counselors, clergy, parents, friends, etc.

GUILT AND THE SINGLE MOTHER

I know this feeling intimately. My son Taylor is, in many ways, unlike other little boys and girls his age. He is different because he is autistic. When I first discovered that Taylor was "different" than other babies, I felt so guilty. "What did I do to create this?" I wondered. "Was it the weight I gained? Was it the long labor I endured?"

Though I had assurances that those situations did not contribute to my son's circumstances, I still felt the guilt. And though he wasn't diagnosed with autism until he was six years old, I had many early years of developmental delays to contend with.

At times, the pain, the grief, and the guilt were more than I felt I could bear. But I soon discovered that my feelings of guilt were getting in the way of my acceptance. I needed to let go of the guilt, realize I wasn't responsible for his autism, and finally move on to deal with the situation.

The same goes for my abilities as a parent. Sometimes I feel like I'm not doing the best job I can. Other times, I feel as if I'm not giving my children enough of my time. But when these feelings arise, I remind myself that time wasted on feeling guilty is time wasted — period.

Guilt does not serve us, it only hinders our growth and freedom to be happy. Whatever your situation, as long as you are diligently doing the best job you can, letting go of guilt will help you to do even better. You can overcome any challenges you encounter, and you can let go of guilt — you just have to work at it harder sometimes than others.

CREEDS FOR MOMMIES TO LIVE BY

- Allow your child to be expressive and creative, encouraging her growth, development and unfoldment.
- Praise and shower your child with compliments. Emphasize her strong points and give far less attention to the rough edges. They'll smooth out over time.
- Never tell your child he is "bad".
- Set an example for your children by being honest, sincere, compassionate, and friendly in all of your affairs so they will mimic integral behavior.
- Where possible, speak kindly to your child of her father; or say little or nothing at all. Your child has the right to love both of you, and should never be made to choose between you, or used as a weapon or spy against the opposite parent.
- Don't expect too much of your child. Don't force him to grow up too quickly. Allow him to be a child.
- Do not make your son your confidant, husband, or replacement "little man". Allow him to be your child.
- Practice patience.
- Talk *to* or *with* your child, and never *down* to him.
- Teach your child respect, and he will be respectful.
- Accept that you are human, and that you will make mistakes. Forgive yourself the mistakes you make. Love and be kind to yourself.

- Be thankful and grateful, reminding yourself often of all that you have.
- Learn from your child to stop and smell the flowers.
- Show your child she can trust you by being dependably consistent in caring and discipline.
- Show your child the love of people, country, and planet, and the joy that comes from helping others.
- Give your child reason to believe she can fulfill her potential and her dreams — and that the world needs what she has to offer.
- Give him plenty of reasons to smile everyday.
- Be kind to your child's mother — she is a very special lady!

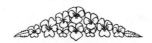

CHAPTER TWELVE

YOUR BABY'S FATHER

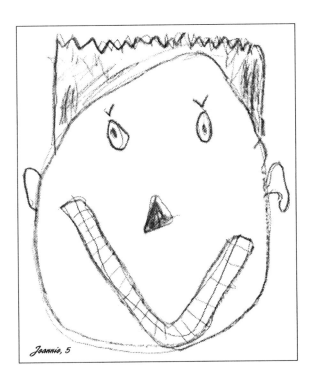

Jeannie, 5

he relationship you have (or do not have) with your baby's father may be one of the more complex issues you face — both during and after your pregnancy. Whether your relationship is good, bad or indifferent, you will undoubtedly experience anxiety where he is concerned.

Because no two situations are the same, I will attempt to cover a spectrum of common dilemmas, questions and problems in this chapter.

DISCUSSING YOUR PREGNANCY WITH YOUR BABY'S FATHER (his rights and yours)

I am not sure I even want to tell "him". Do I have a legal obligation to do so?

While you have no legal obligation to tell your child's biological father that you are pregnant, several questions remain: Do you have a moral obligation to tell him? Does he have a right to know? Does your child have a right to know his father?

Unless the man is a clear danger to you or your child, it is wise to consider these questions carefully. The choice you make today will deeply affect the lives of many people besides yourself for many years to come. In addition to the father, this decision makes a "choice" for the grandparents, aunts, uncles, and others. Perhaps more importantly, it makes a choice for your baby. Are you prepared to be responsible for that choice?

While telling the father–to–be may open up a can of worms you'd just as soon avoid, your secret may catch up to you one day. You may have to deal with the fall–out later on. Furthermore, not telling him does not guarantee that he will not find out sooner than later. If he does, he would be entitled to assert his legal rights to see the child (or even seek custody) if he so desired.

Nobody can make this choice for you, but you should give it careful consideration before you decide to keep his child from him.

I'm not sure how he's going to react to the news.

You'd be surprised how many women expect one reaction from their partner and get another. There's just no way to predict how he's going to react. Some women find their mates to be more responsive than they expected. Others assume that because the relationship is good, they won't get a negative reaction — but this is not always the case.

While your pregnancy is causing all kinds of changes in you, your partner will accept or reject the news based upon how he perceives a child will change *his* life. His considerations will likely be about the responsibilities and expense of raising a child. And he may worry about giving up his freedom. He may feel too young or too old to have a child. He may or may not be willing to talk about these things.

Unless you know for sure that he wants to have a child with you, there's not a "best way" to give him the news. But it is probably better to tell him in private. Approach him when he is in a calm, agreeable mood. Don't tell him just before he has an important meeting or is preoccupied with other things. And be gentle in your approach. If he's not initially elated, try and give him some time to digest the news.

I am so hurt. I just told my boyfriend that I was pregnant and he told me he doesn't want any part of it. What are his responsibilities?

While the courts can compel him to take a paternity test, and to pay child support, (See Establishing Paternity and Child Support in Chapter 13 for more detailed information), they cannot force this man to be a part of your child's life.

It may be preferable to you and your child that the father participate in your child's life. However, if he's not interested, you can try to change his mind; but there may not be much else you can do. The sooner you accept this, the better off you will be on an emotional level. If Dad does not choose to be a part of your child's life, you and your child will be the ones that need to make the adjustments to accept and adjust to this.

If your partner has expressed his intentions to be an absent father, you are probably feeling a lot of emotions right now, especially if his reaction is a surprise to you. You may be feeling vulnerable, sad or even angry. Rejection from the man you love can be deeply disappointing — even devastating.

While I know from experience that it may be hard to take the focus off of "him" right now, it will help you if you put your energies into a healthy and happy pregnancy. You will be wasting the beautiful experience of your pregnancy if you are so possessed by him and what he's going to do that you do not focus on yourself and your developing baby.

In time, he may just come around.

In time, the guy just may come around. But pushing or threatening him isn't going to make it happen. Instead, surround yourself with loving friends and family. Keep busy. Eat healthily, exercise, and do nice things for yourself to keep your mind off of him as much as possible.

My baby's father treated me badly during my pregnancy. But now that the baby is here, he wants to be involved. I'm still angry and don't know what to do.

Many of the mothers I interviewed had this experience. I call it the "Little Red Hen" scenario. He wasn't there to help you bake the bread, but now he wants to eat it.

It can be frustrating when you are torn between conflicting emotions. You want him to be a part of your life, and/or your child's life, but you're still angry.

Now you have to make a choice. Are you going to hold on to the anger and let it creep into your relationship over and over? You may be tempted to punish him for his lack of support during your pregnancy. After all, you may be thinking...he should pay for the shabby way he treated you! But will that bring you the happiness you truly desire? Is it in yours, and your child's best interest to stay angry?

If you can't get over it but he truly wants to make amends and start over, you might suggest some counseling to help you get through it (and over it) together. A good mediator can help you to explore and resolve your feelings when they're too confused to sort through on your own.

Respect yourself.

If he doesn't want any part of this child, demands that you have an abortion, or breaks up with you over your pregnancy, try to avoid ugly scenes. You are better than that! Begging and pleading with him will probably not change his mind. And having an abortion (if you don't choose it for yourself) just because he wants you to, will hurt you in a lasting way.

Respect yourself. Love yourself enough to let him go. You deserve a man who cherishes you and your child. But first you must cherish yourself.

My ex is abusive, and I am afraid he will harm my child. What can I do to prevent this?

If your child's father has abused you, or you suspect he may abuse your child, consult with an attorney immediately. The attorney can advise you about legal remedies and, depending upon the circumstances, help you to attempt to obtain a court order of protection against him. (In some states, you can go to the courthouse on your own to apply for a domestic violence injunction).

Depending upon the circumstances, a court may order supervised visitation, or no visitation at all. If you are successful in obtaining a protective order, or domestic violence injunction, and he is still living in the home, the order will force him to leave the home and stay away from you and your child. Such an order will not have any bearing upon his financial obligation to support his child.

If you are in an abusive or life–threatening situation, it is particularly important for you to seek help. Call a private attorney, Legal Aid Society (or the police if the threat is immediate). Call information for the number of a battered women's shelter in your area, or contact you local YWCA for assistance. If you have a social worker, contact him or her immediately.

Whatever you do, get out of this dangerous and potentially life–

threatening situation. You have a responsibility to yourself and to your child to do so.

A word of caution with respect to this issue: it is unfortunate, but some women (and men) will use issues such as domestic violence as a weapon against an ex partner, when the fact is, there exists no threat or act of violence. If the act or threat of violence is not real, *never* use this as a way to get back at, intimidate, or gain leverage over your child's father.

"WHO IS MY DADDY?"

WHEN DADDY DOESN'T COME TO SEE YOUR CHILD

If your child's biological father is not involved in her life on an active and consistent basis, it is inevitable thet she will one day ask: "Who is my Daddy?", "Why doesn't my Daddy come to see me?", "Why doesn't my Daddy love me?", or any variation on these questions.

At some point your child will begin to understand that many other kids have two parents but she doesn't. On Father's Day, when the other kids are making presents for daddy at school, she may feel different, deprived and left–out. Perhaps the kids down the block will play ball outside with their father — as your son looks longingly at this event and wonders why his daddy isn't around to play ball with him.

Coming to terms with daddy's absence can be a confusing time for a child. While some children appear to take this issue in stride, others feel outwardly or inwardly angry, sad or resentful that daddy doesn't come to visit.

Asking questions about daddy is normal and healthy. It's important for your child to feel safe enough to express her feelings and ask questions. In anticipation of this likely event, you might want to give some thought to what you are going to tell your child.

Thinking it through in advance will help put you in touch with your own feelings and sort out what is most appropriate to convey to your child. Otherwise, when put on the spot, you may not be able to answer your child's questions as effectively as you would if you had prepared for them in advance.

Whatever the reasons that your child's father does not participate in her life, as her mother, they are undoubtedly very sensitive issues for you. As mothers we want our children to have everything they need. You may never be able to provide her with her real daddy, and this may bring up strong feelings for you. Guilt, anger and resentment are not uncommon emotions for mothers to have when the father does not maintain a relationship with his child. His absence will affect your child's emotions, self–esteem and relationship to the world.

How do I approach talking to my child about her father?

Psychologists tell us that it is very important and necessary when questions about missing fathers arise, that we answer them honestly and at an age–appropriate level. Obviously a four or five year old is not ready to hear the same amount of detail that a nine, ten or eleven year old is ready to hear. Attempt to talk to your child at a level that matches her comprehension. Consider carefully how much information she can absorb and understand.

How much detail should I give my child?

When you begin your talk, be sensitive to your child's feelings. Try to be as honest as possible and keep your answers simple and direct. While you may choose to omit certain facts and some gritty details, you should not lie to your child or make up stories about his father and his whereabouts. Not only does lying send messages to your child about your own morals and character, but it disrespects your child's intelligence and his right to know the truth. Children can sense when we're not being honest. Additionally, any lie you tell today may very well come back to haunt you (and your child) in the future.

The respect you show your child by discussing the matter in a straight–forward manner will contribute to the overall tone of your relationship with him. Remember, trust between a parent and child is vital, and you need to establish a trusting relationship early on. This includes the way in which you handle this particular issue.

From your child's perspective, it doesn't really matter who left whom, who wanted the baby and who didn't, who abandoned the child, who was wrong or right, etc. These are all irrelevant issues for a young child. Such details are better left to yourself. It is important to avoid "trashing" your child's father by speaking negatively about him. Even overhearing a telephone conversation where you are discussing "his problems" can do damage to a child.

A child's good opinion of both parents is very important to his or her own self–perception and development. We do not want to create fairytales, but we do not want to hurt our children with real or imagined "bad guy" stories about their fathers either. No matter how much you may dislike or disrespect him, you should never emphasize this to your child — directly or indirectly. You can get those feelings off your chest privately with friends or a good therapist.

Your child is a reflection of both parents.

If you emphasize negative thoughts and feelings about your child's father, it is very likely that your child will, on some level, take it personally. Children see themselves as a reflection of both of their parents. When angry, negative or hostile information is imparted to your child about her opposite parent, it will often leave her with questions, feelings and insecurities about herself. These emotions can leave lasting impressions and scars that do not heal. To say to a child "You're just like your father!" in an angry or negative way, is hurtful and potentially damaging.

Children tend to personalize the world around them, and may blame themselves for not being worthy of their father's love and attention. On a deep level, a child may feel that if daddy is bad, then she must be bad too. This can set the stage for a child to develop mistrust and resentments; and may well affect the relationships she enters into as an adult.

Emphasize the positive qualities of your child's father.

It is important for you to emphasize to your child the positive and terrific things about her father. If you are lucky enough to have a good relationship with her father, and you parted on amicable terms, that obviously makes it easier to relate positive stories and impressions to your child. But even if you parted on unfriendly terms, you can still manage to find good qualities to talk about. Even if you cannot see anything positive about your child's father, if you look at what attracted you to him in the first place, you are likely to come up with something.

Try to remember and retell these impressions. Surely he has *some* good qualities. Focus on his strengths, skills, abilities, intelligence, talents, etc. Share these positive attributes and qualities with your child. Let her know the positive ways she takes after her father. Give her a sense of pride in her heritage.

You have a great deal of influence over your child's feelings and beliefs. Thus, you can help her to see the light or lead her into darkness. Even in the most difficult situation, if we try hard enough, we can choose to make lemonade out of lemons. And if you try hard enough, I'm sure you can find some nice qualities about your child's father to share with her.

Hopefully you have established a good rapport with your ex. If you haven't, remember, that your child is the important one here. You want to help her to understand and accept her circumstances and herself.

My child is deeply hurt over her father's absence. What can I do?

When there is pain and hurt over this issue, it makes things even more difficult to deal with — for both of you. As a loving parent, it is your natural instinct to want to fix things; to make them all better; to make problems go away. As nurturers, most mothers would do anything to protect their child.

Unfortunately, in this situation we cannot fully protect our children against the loss or absence of a natural father. This is the reality and it really hurts.

As tempting as it may seem, you cannot help or protect your child by avoiding this issue. You must deal with it. Not to do so will only make the problem bigger later on. And eventually in one form or another it will come up again.

Your child should feel free to express her feelings.

Your child needs to feel secure and understood. And she needs to know that she is free to talk openly and honestly about her feelings. Telling her you don't want to talk about her dad may damage her ability to learn to express her feelings.

Keep in mind that you also send a message to your child that it's not safe to talk about certain things by what you *do not* say. While this issue may be painful for you, imagine what is going through her little head. She needs to know it's okay to express any anger or sadness she feels. She especially needs your love and support to help her accept the situation as it is, and to understand that she is not to blame.

Keep the lines of communication open — and encourage your son or daughter to talk about their feelings. In this way, you can help to soften the blow of an absent father. However, if your child displays serious bouts of depression or inappropriate behavior over this issue, it would be wise to consult a professional who is trained to deal with such problems.

There are no guarantees how your child will react.

In observing numerous children and adults I have known who have had absent parents, I have come to see that there is no guarantee as to how a child will handle this issue. There are many factors that play into the equation. Thus, every child will react differently according to his or her circumstances and temperament; as well as the mother's attitude. While one child appears to handle the absence of one parent very well and is able to come to terms with the problem, another may suffer short or long–term emotional pain.

Cushioning the blow.

In addition to encouraging open communication, another way to help your child come to terms with his loss is to provide a stable home environment and positive male role models. Your child will handle dad's absence more easily if he is secure, if his home life is stable, and if he can count on special relationships to be there for him.

The adults I have known who were successfully raised by single–parents seemed to deal with the loss or absence of a parent best when they had a solid foundation of love, nurturing and support. When open and honest communication was available to them, they were more likely to grow up to feel secure and happy.

Conversely, the children and adults who were adversely affected over the absence of one parent, were more likely to be children who were neglected; emotionally or physically abused; made to feel unimportant; told that their "father was a jerk"; and discouraged from self–expression at home — among other negative and dysfunctional conditions. Any combination of these factors, even in a two–parent home, creates misery for a child.

If you are having difficulty dealing with the loss of your partner, if you feel unable to effectively communicate with your child about him, or if you tend to communicate negativity or hostility to your child, you may want to consider obtaining professional help to guide you through the rough spots. A good counselor or therapist can help you to deal with your own reactions, so that you can more effectively deal with your child regarding these issues.

If you feel that your child is not handling the loss or separation from his father very well, a professional who is trained to deal with your child's feelings can greatly help to improve the situation for both of you. You can receive counseling separately or together.

DROP–IN DADS

In my situation, my eldest son's father is, for the most part, an absentee father who sees his son on an infrequent basis. This was okay for the first four years of Taylor's life when he did not understand what was happening. However, as Taylor grew older, the drop–in father routine seemed to do more harm than good. Dad's irresponsible behavior sent mixed messages to our little boy — who was both confused and hurt over his father's behavior.

When Taylor was six years old, he began to create fantasies about his daddy coming to take him to lunch and to amusement parks. In fact, Taylor's fantasies were so real, I thought he actually spoke to his father on the telephone. But for nearly a year, his daddy never came.

When Taylor asked me (over and over) where his father was, I would tell him that his father was "busy". But that didn't stop Taylor from being deeply hurt and disappointed — in fact, it only seemed to prolong the pain.

Over time, it occurred to me that I was telling half–truths to Taylor and as long as I did this, Taylor would hold on to "false" hope — only to eventually be let down again and again.

I had been struggling with the balance of being honest with Taylor and my mother–lion protection instincts. There were times I wanted to say to Taylor "Sorry baby, your father moved away to a foreign country and didn't leave his telephone number!" — but I knew I couldn't do that to him.

Finally, I consulted several psychologists and friends about the problem. They all told me that Taylor needed to know the truth. So I decided that the next time Taylor asked about his daddy, I would tell him the truth.

A few weeks later, when Taylor brought up his dad again, I took a deep breath and told him that his daddy did not want to see him at that point in time, and that he *wasn't* coming to see him. I told him that I loved him so much that I wanted him the moment I found out that he was in my tummy; but that his father didn't feel the same way.

I let Taylor know that it wasn't *him* his daddy didn't want to see — but that his daddy just wasn't prepared to have *any* child at all. As I talked to Taylor, I was very careful not to speak negatively about his father. I kept our conversation brief, and let him ask the questions he had on his mind.

That conversation was one of the most difficult I have ever had in my life. And it broke my heart to see the look in Taylor's eyes. When he protested "My daddy is too coming!", I turned to my desperate child and said: "No baby, your daddy isn't coming — he's really not coming." I turned away so he wouldn't see my tears. I didn't want Taylor to think that *he* had made me cry.

Sometimes, the truth hurts.

Having been so blunt with Taylor may seem like a radical approach. But not telling him would not have served him either. Eventually, he was going to understand anyway. So too, will your child. While you may want to leave out the more complex or painful details, the harsh truth is better than unanswered questions and lingering hope.

Many of the mothers I interviewed told me that they experienced similar frustrations with the problems of drop–in dads. Cara, a single mother of two children said: "What can I do? If I attempt to protect my child by telling his father to stay away, then I'm the "bad–guy". And besides, he probably wouldn't listen to me anyway. On the other hand, if I don't put my foot down and put an end to the problem, I'm not protecting my child. Either way, my child suffers."

For many of us, dad's irresponsible behavior puts us in the hot seat. We must deal with the aftermath of disappointment when daddy doesn't come back for a long stretch of time. And yet, as Cara pointed out, we're the "bad guy" if we put our foot down and say "no more!" Unfortunately, the court's can't help with this situation, because they can't legislate morality and diligent parenting.

There's no easy answer.

It's not always easy to find the best words to comfort our children and honestly answer their questions. It is especially hard to try to explain why daddy doesn't come around. But it's your job to try.

There could be a thousand different reasons why dad isn't available. Maybe dad really is a jerk. Perhaps he is abusive; and an undesirable role model. Or maybe he is just lost and afraid to face up to his responsibilities. It's unfortunate, but dad's problems have become yours and your child's problems.

When your child hurts over this issue, it hurts you. This is one of the toughest issues for single mothers to deal with. Your awareness and gentle, loving approach in answering your child's questions is important. So is expert advice — so when in doubt, seek it out.

For those of you who brought your child into this world through artificial insemination; and for those who do not know who the father is, while you won't be dealing with a drop–in dad, if your child's father doesn't visit regularly, you will still need to face this issue at one point or another.

Dealing with the issue of an absent father is a delicate situation which has no easy answers. When things get tough, you just have to love your kids extra hard, talk with them about their feelings, try to be strong for them, and pray. Using any or all of the exercises in this books will also help.

MITIGATING THE DAMAGE –
FINDING A MENTOR FOR YOUR CHILD

Your child's ability to cope with the absence of her biological father also has a lot to do with your efforts to provide her with an extended family which includes good and positive male role models. Your own father, brothers, uncles, and male friends are sometimes good places to start. Perhaps her father's family will choose to be involved.

There are also a variety of other places you can look to find terrific male role models, including your church or synagogue (try posting an ad on the bulletin board for a "big brother" or "big sister"). Or, perhaps a man in your workplace will be willing to mentor your child.

Many wonderful organizations exist which are designed especially for kids. Brownies, Girl Scouts, Cub Scouts, Boy Scouts, etc., are excellent organizations, and are helpful in getting your kids involved in a variety of fun, positive, goal oriented, fun activities.

For other child–oriented organizations, look in your yellow pages under the heading "Child Development Centers". Churches, local parks and recreation, YMCA and YWCA also offer terrific low–cost programs for kids.

BIG BROTHERS, BIG SISTERS OF AMERICA

Big Brothers, Big Sisters is the largest network of mentoring organizations serving children, families and communities in the United States. It cites more than 500 agencies in all 50 states. Founded in 1904, Big Brothers, Big Sisters matches adult volunteers with school–aged children from primarily single–parent homes. Big Brothers and Big Sisters (Bigs) serve as mentors and role models to their Little Brothers and Little Sisters (Littles). The volunteers commit to several hours weekly for a minimum of one year. The friendships are supported by a professionally–staffed agency and case managers.

The relationships which are developed between Bigs and Littles provide the children with an increased sense of belonging, enhanced communication skills, and improved performance at school, at home and in the community. In a study conducted in 1992 and 1993, research indicated that a child with a Big Brother or Big Sister was 46% less likely to begin using illegal drugs; 27% less likely to begin using alcohol; 52% less likely to skip school; and 37% less likely to skip a class. Littles are more confident in their schoolwork; less likely to hit someone; and they got along better with their families.

The screening and matching of Bigs and Littles is an in–depth process. Men and women who are interested in becoming Bigs are put through a very detailed, psychological evaluation intended to screen out men and women who are undesirable or potentially harmful to a child. Extensive background checks are performed, including review of police records.

Unfortunately, there can often be a waiting period of several months (or longer) before a match is made, as there are not enough Big Brothers and Big Sisters to go around. The service is free. However, Big Brothers, Big Sisters is a non–profit organization so it encourages mothers to donate time to fundraising efforts, if at all possible.

To find out more about Big Brothers, Big Sisters, contact your local BB/BS agency listed in the white pages of the telephone directory, or call the National Office of Big Brothers, Big Sisters of America at (215) 567–7000.

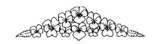

—CHAPTER THIRTEEN—

MORE LEGAL ISSUES

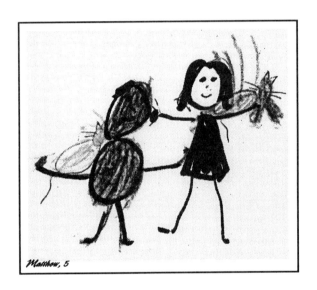

Matthew, 5

ESTABLISHING PATERNITY

What is paternity?

Paternity means fatherhood. Establishing paternity means that a Judge/Commissioner signs a court order officially identifying the legal father.

Why is establishing paternity important?

IDENTITY: A child has the right to know his or her parents. This knowledge may also be necessary in the future to prevent your child from marrying a close relative.

INHERITANCE: Your child has a right of inheritance from both parents. Your child also has rights to other benefits both parents may have which might include Social Security, medical, and veteran's benefits. Getting these benefits are easier when paternity is legally established.

MEDICAL: Your child needs to know if she may have inherited any disease or disorders, many of which may not be detected at birth or in childhood.

MONEY: Both parents have a legal obligation to support their children — even if the pregnancy was unintentional. Children who are supported by only one parent, often do not have enough money for their needs.

RESPONSIBILITY: The father has the right to know and the responsibility to support his child — and you have the right to get help and support from the father in raising your child.

When should I establish paternity?

You may start the proceeding as soon as you find out you are pregnant. If he denies being the father and blood tests are required, you will have to wait for the blood test until after the baby is born. However, if you have to wait for this procedure, in the meantime, you can immediately ask the court to order a blood test, payment of support and/or medical expenses. It is important to start as early as possible because child support may be ordered back to the date you filed with the court.

Who can establish paternity?

Either the mother, the father, or the child can do this procedure, even after the child turns 18. However, if the child is over the age of 18, it may limit your ability to collect child support. If you and the father are in agreement, you can do this procedure together.

My partner wants to acknowledge his child and help me raise her. Can we establish paternity without a blood test?

Yes. After your baby is born, the hospital will provide you with an Acknowledgment of Paternity form. This form can also be obtained from any Child Support Enforcement Office. This form protects you, your child, and the father. It establishes the baby's legal father, protects your child's inheritance and other legal rights, and establishes your right to collect child support. It also protects the father's right to see his child.

If he denies my baby is his, how do I go about establishing paternity?

If the father is not willing to sign an Acknowledgment of Paternity form, you will have to file a lawsuit. Contact a lawyer, legal clinic, Legal Aid Society, or your local City or District Attorney's office. You will be asked to provide information related to your pregnancy and the name of the person your believe is the father.

Will I have to answer personal questions about my relationship with my child's father?

Yes, although the questions aren't meant to embarrass you. Nonetheless, they are often necessary to establish that you had a relationship with the alleged father which resulted in the birth of your child.

My baby's father and I are living together. Why should I establish paternity?

It's a good idea to establish paternity under any circumstances in order to prevent potential future problems. Though the father may agree to help you now, he may change his mind later on. This may make it more difficult to establish paternity, particularly if the father moves away.

Furthermore, if the father dies and paternity has not been legally established, you may not be able to prove your child's entitlement to Social Security Survivor benefits, inheritance, life insurance, etc.

What if I'm not sure who the father is?

If you are unsure because you had a relationship with more than one man around the time of conception, the court may require that all possible fathers have their blood tested. Based on the results of the tests and other evidence, the court will determine paternity.

Blood testing.

If a man denies that he is the biological father of a child, a court may use the results of blood testing in making a determination of paternity. However, because some courts do not consider the results of such testing to render a finding of paternity as a scientific certainty, blood testing is not used to automatically prove paternity — but rather, only to show the likelihood that a man cannot be excluded in the population as the minor child's biological father. This is an important point, because, for example, while a blood test may come back at 98% paternity, this does not mean that the court will find that the tested individual *is* the father.

For purposes of the court proceeding, it may only be used as one supporting factor for the court to find that the individual is the father. While in some jurisdictions blood tests can raise a presumption of paternity, they may not necessarily establish paternity itself. Nonetheless, in almost all circumstances, a blood test which comes back at such a high percentage of probability will create the child support obligation.

Types of Blood Testing.

There are two different types of blood testing — HLA and DNA. DNA is considered to be more accurate, and can be administered upon a child at birth. Additionally, the DNA method requires that less blood be drawn than the HLA method. The HLA method cannot be administered until the baby is at least six months old.

In any case, blood testing will compare blood types, tissue types, and genetic profiles and will establish, within a reasonable certainty, a link (or lack thereof) between the child and the father.

Once the court has determined through the use of blood testing that the man is most certain to be the child's father, he has no legal recourse to continue to deny parentage or to escape his legal obligation to the child. In other words, he can deny he is the father, but that will not dismiss his legal, financial obligation to your child.

What other evidence is helpful in establishing paternity?

There are many things which may be used as evidence in a paternity hearing (though they do not, in and of themselves, prove paternity). Among those things are: The father has told others that he is the father; he claims a tax deduction; he declared the child on his health insurance; he agreed to be named on the birth certificate; he supported the child financially; he admits to sexual relations with you at the time of conception; or he visits your child regularly, or sends cards/letters, etc., to the child.

CHILD SUPPORT

Whether you have decided to seek child support or not, it is prudent for you to have a basic understanding of how the laws concerning this issue work. It will be helpful if you consult with an attorney to better understand how child support works in your particular jurisdiction so as not to shortchange yourself. Additionally, it is advisable to consider and address issues of health insurance, uncovered health expenses for the minor child, as well as life insurance for one or both of the parents for security in the event of death of either party.

I can't afford a private attorney. Who can I turn to?

If you need help locating the father and/or collecting child support — and can't afford a private attorney — contact your local Office of Child Support Enforcement. To request a free Child Support Enforcement Information Package, write to: Administration for Children and Families, Office of Child Support Enforcement, Department of Health & Human Services, 378 L'Enfant Promenade SW, Washington, DC 20447, or call (202) 401–9383.

If your income is low enough to qualify you for Aid to Families with Dependent Children (AFDC), they will help you find the father if he has disappeared, and help you collect child support. To locate the AFDC office in your area, look under Social Services Department, Social and Health Services, or similar heading in your phone book.

You can also call your local Legal Aid Society or Foundation to determine if you are eligible for Legal Aid assistance. Legal Aid was established to make sure that the poor have access to the justice system in civil legal matters.

Though each Legal Aid Society/Foundation's services vary, they generally provide free counsel, representation, advocacy and community education in the areas of housing, government benefits, family (including child custody and support disputes), consumer, immigration and employment law, among other things. If they will not take your case, contact your local county or district attorneys office — or the attorney general of your jurisdiction. These agencies are listed in your yellow pages under the heading "State Government".

If the father of your child fails to meet his child support obligations, another organization you can contact is The Association for Children for Enforcement of Support, Inc. (ACES). This national, non–profit organization is dedicated to assisting disadvantaged children affected by parents who fail to meet legal and moral child support obligations. They offer educational, advocacy, outreach, and counseling programs.

Additionally, monthly chapter meetings for discussion and problem solving often include guest speakers from child support agencies as well as professionals such as attorneys and judges. They also distribute printed information about state and federal child support laws, legal rights and methods. For more information, contact ACES hotline at (800) 537–7072, or call their national headquarters at (419) 472–0047.

For additional referrals, see the Resource Section at the back of this book.

Be patient. Expect your case to take some time.

While you do not pay for many of these public services, the process can be painfully slow and it can take months or even years before you receive your first check. Be prepared to be patient, and be sure to make periodic telephone calls to the agency handling your case to monitor progress.

It will help if you are able to give them important information about your baby's father. This includes his complete name; driver's license and social security numbers; last known address and telephone number (home and work); employment information; date of birth; county or state of birth; mother's first and maiden names; father's first and last names; bank and/or credit card account numbers; and any other pertinent information you may have about him.

My child's father lives in another state. How can I collect child support?

Although each state has its own guidelines, rules, policies, and avenues of enforcement, there are certain federal laws which govern throughout the United States. Because the individual state support laws were found to be non–uniform and chaotic, the Uniform Reciprocal Enforcement of Support Act (URESA) was enacted.

URESA is state legislation which has been uniformly adopted throughout the states in all jurisdictions. URESA is legislation intended to enforce child support and enforcement when the parents reside in different states.

Under URESA, the Petitioner (in this case, the mother) requesting support files a petition in her home state. The petition may include previous orders of the court in her state or even another state; may state that the child needing support lives with the Petitioner; or it may even be an initial action for paternity.

After the papers are filed, the initiating state sends the documentation and petition to the state where the Respondent (in this case, the father) resides. Another court action is initiated in the second state where the father is sued for support. If the father denies paternity, blood tests can be ordered through the URESA action.

When parents are unmarried, does the father have a legal obligation to support his child?

In general, the law provides that the father *and* mother of a child have an equal responsibility to support and educate their child in the manner suitable to the child's circumstances — taking into consideration the respective earnings or earning capacities of the parents and their standard of living. Usually, the parent who has physical custody of the child or children is entitled to receive child support from the other parent.

While it is your right to decide to bear the financial responsibilities of raising your child without monetary assistance from your child's father, it is also your right to receive child support for your minor child. It does not matter whether you were or were not married to the baby's father. When you have custody of your minor child, your child's natural father is not excused from paying child support simply because he was not married to you when the baby was conceived. The law in the United States is very clear on this issue: the natural father of your minor child has a legal obligation to make child support payments.

An amicable approach.

Hopefully, you and your child's father can come to a reasonable and amicable settlement that works well for the three of you. That's certainly easier for everyone. If you can reach such a mutually acceptable agreement without the need to drag the matter through the courts, I would urge you to do so. Family law attorneys are generally very expensive, and a court battle can be quite lengthy. Moreover, a fight in court can get very ugly and cause a great deal of pain for everyone involved.

Mediation.

If you and your child's father are unable to make any progress on your own, one way to avoid going to court is to agree to attend mediation. However, mediation is a voluntary process, and thus both parties must agree to attend.

A mediator is a trained counselor. The mediator can be a professional mediator, a family law attorney, a member of the clergy, or a family counselor. Oftentimes, attorneys make the best mediators because they are armed with the law concerning child support, health insurance, life insurance, as well as other potential issues including those of visitation and shared parental responsibility.

The mediator is not a judge, and will not advise or make any decisions for either party. Mediation is not a substitute for obtaining legal advice. It is a mediator's role to help the parties work out an amicable resolution.

A mediator is basically an impartial referee who oversees the settlement negotiations between the parties. Once you come to an agreement concerning the issues of child support, custody and visitation, generally it is then simply a matter of formality to get the court to approve the agreement between the parties. You should note here, however, that a court can alter your arrangement if it determines in its discretion that the support is inadequate or that the child's best interest is not served. The court always has the final authority to approve your agreement.

Along these lines, it is important to understand that any agreement worked out between you and the father of your child which is not approved by the court (reduced to an order or judgment), will not be enforceable through contempt or other means if the father stops making his payments. Be sure to get a court order or judgment on any agreement worked out between you.

For more information on mediation, call the Academy of Family Mediators at (617) 674-2663 for a list of mediators in your state, or the Children's Rights Council at (800) 787-4KIDS. You can also check your yellow pages under the heading "Mediation Services", or contact your local family law court to see if they can refer you to someone in your area.

We've tried to work it out between us, but we just don't agree. What do I do now?

If you and your child's father cannot mutually agree upon the issue of child support, and you have exhausted all efforts to work out a settlement between you, a court of law will have to decide the issue. The question now becomes: "How do I proceed?" There are several ways you can approach the task of collecting child support through the courts.

FINDING A FAMILY LAW ATTORNEY.

The best way to proceed is to hire a qualified, experienced attorney who specializes in the area of family law. In attempting to find someone who will "go to bat for you", it is recommended that you interview several lawyers before you make your decision. An attorney may or may not charge you a consultation fee for an initial meeting. Be sure to ask prior to your first meeting. Referrals from friends, or from your local or state bar association, are good ways to find an attorney.

What questions should I ask a prospective attorney?

- How long have you been a family law specialist?
- Do you have sufficient time to devote to my case?
- What is your hourly rate (or flat fee)?
- What can I expect the costs to be? (costs are different than fees, and include filing fees, deposition costs, service of process, subpoenas, mediation costs, messenger, fax charges, long distance telephone calls, etc.)
- Do you require a retainer fee to be paid in advance? How much?
- In what increments do you bill for telephone calls?
- Will you be responsible for handling my case (making appearances, etc.), or will you have associates and/or paralegals working on the matter?
- What are the merits of my case and how will you proceed?

As you talk, you will get a feel for this attorney's demeanor and attitudes. Is the attorney confident, professional, and well spoken? Do you feel comfortable with them? If you do not get a good feeling from them, it would be wise to move on and look for someone else. Trust your instincts.

My new attorney asked me to sign a retainer agreement. What is this document?

A retainer, or fee agreement, is a written agreement between you and the attorney which sets forth the terms of your legal representation. The document is intended to protect you as well as the attorney. It should set forth the attorneys hourly rate, the hourly rate of any associates or paralegals who will work on your case, and any retainer amount to be paid. It should also explain what costs are paid in addition to the hourly or flat fee.

Your attorney should fully explain the intent and content of the agreement to you. If you have any questions, or don't understand a particular provision, feel free to ask them about it *prior* to signing your name to any agreement.

Speculating on the cost of the case.

While your attorney can speculate on the expected cost of your proceedings, there is really no way to determine exactly how long your case will take, or exactly how much it will cost to resolve. Unless your attorney is charging you a flat fee, he or she can only guess how much you will ultimately pay for legal services.

Your child's father can, and may, for good reasons, or as a tactical advantage, tie you up with delay after delay through the court system. Unfortunately, these delays can run your legal bill through the roof. But within the law, many delays are legal and to be expected.

In other instances, a court can bump a case to make room for another, or take the matter off its docket/calendar for any number of reasons — causing additional delays. And if your attorney has already traveled to the court to make the appearance, you will likely be billed for the time and travel anyway. There are a number of reasons your fees and costs may become unexpectedly high.

While costs may be high, many jurisdictions may allow you to seek costs and attorneys fees against the father. However, though a court may ultimately determine that the father should pay a portion or all of your legal fees, I wouldn't suggest you take it for granted that you will be reimbursed. It doesn't always happen that way.

How much do lawyers charge per hour?

The hourly rates for attorneys vary significantly from city to city and state to state. Hourly rates range from between approximately $100.00 to $400.00 per hour depending upon where you live, but the average rates are approximately $125.00 to $250.00 per hour. However, some attorneys (especially in today's economy) may charge a flat fee. Attorneys will often work out a payment schedule with you and some even accept credit cards.

What about legal centers or clinics?

You can find referrals to local legal clinics by looking in your phone book under the listing "Legal Clinics". Many of the clinics offer low–cost legal services. Others are attorney–assisted legal centers, where you can represent yourself — but an attorney will assist you to navigate through the legal system.

This method is called "In propria persona", "pro per", or "pro se". You will be assisted in handling your own case, purchasing court forms, learning filing procedures, etc.

If, however, all of the issues are not amicably resolved between the two of you, or if the father is represented by private counsel, handling your own case is not advised. There is a saying "An attorney who represents him(her)self, has a fool for a client" — and in this case you'll likely get what you pay for.

Paralegals.

Another possibility is to hire a paralegal. A paralegal is not licensed to practice law but is trained to aid lawyers. An attorney should oversee the process, but the paralegal will do the footwork. This is a less expensive route because you are being charged rates for paralegal services and not the hourly rates of an attorney.

Generally, there is a set fee to file a petition and obtain a Financial Affidavit or Income and Expense Declaration from your child's father. A Financial Affidavit or Income and Expense Declaration is a document prepared by each party which states the amount of money you each make and spend. It is used to help determine the amount of child support to be paid.

Additionally, many states now require mandatory disclosure of certain documents including income tax returns, pay stubs, K1s, W–2s, 1099's, copies of recent loan applications, financial statements, and copies of any other documents reflecting income. The purpose of requiring these documents is to insure against fraud of one party understating income on the financial affidavit. Whether disclosure is mandatory or not, you should request these documents. A paralegal will help you get this information from the father.

The range for paralegal services varies, but you can expect to pay approximately $50 per hour. Additionally, you will pay costs, including filing fees and process service fees. Paralegals can be found in the yellow pages under the heading "Paralegals".

A word of caution when hiring legal clinics or paralegals:

Family law specialist Jonathan Zahler cautions: "I do not recommend legal clinics or paralegals handling cases. In 99% of cases that have crossed my desk wherein a paralegal or legal clinic was involved in the paperwork, they have completely missed several issues, determined child support and other issues incorrectly, and have had only quasi–enforceable agreements. At the same time, they have absolutely no professional liability or responsibility for their actions." In Zahler's opinion, paralegals and legal clinics were invented in response to the old adage: "Penny wise and pound foolish".

Zahler recommends that if you must resort to a legal clinic or paralegal, you should be absolutely certain that an attorney is overseeing the work — not just in name, but in actuality — and that the attorney is ultimately responsible for the result.

Guidelines for determining the amount of support.

Each state has its own guidelines for determining the amount of support that is to be paid, though the amount is also contingent upon individual circumstances. Child support is most often determined by the supporting parent (in this case the father's) income — or, in some cases, the amount he is capable of earning.

Other determining factors will be the individual needs of the child. If your child has special needs (i.e., a handicap, special education needs, medical needs, child care, etc.), the court may also consider these circumstances.

If your child's father is not working, a court may order him to pay support based on what he would be earning at a full–time job at at least the applicable minimum wage, and higher if he is capable of earning more. If his income increases in the future, you must go back to court to request to change the support amount.

However, in many cases you will not know if the father's income increases or decreases in the future. The only way for you to find out is to file a lawsuit for change of child support and conduct "evidentiary discovery" on the income. And in some cases, if the father's income has decreased, the court will decrease the amount of support he pays.

As you can see, in attempting to obtain child support, you will often run into snags and delays along the way. You may need to hire a private investigator to do an asset check to determine the father's ability to pay, or to find him if he has disappeared. You must be able to have legal papers served personally upon him, and you must know where he is in order to do this. Yet another potential set–back, may be contested paternity.

I have a court order for child support, but the father isn't in compliance.

Even after an order is granted by the court, another difficulty many women run into is collecting child support.

Just because the court determines a weekly, semi–weekly, monthly or semi–monthly amount that is to be paid for support of the child does not mean that the support will be paid on time or at all.

Many fathers will directly disobey a court order. They may even move out of state or leave the country to attempt to avoid their legal obligations.

Ultimately, if the father is not complying with a court order, the court has the power to enforce the support in several ways: Contempt for non–payment is often punishable by sanctions (a penalty for breaking the law) and/or by Wage Assignment, Withholding Order, or Income Deduction Order. Such assignment or order causes support monies to be withheld directly from the father's paycheck –– and often makes provisions for back, unpaid support. Most, if not all states, use some for of registry on depository for collecting child support from the father's employer and for keeping records of payments.

You should get a Wage Assignment, Withholding Order, or Income Deduction Order even if your child's father is not presently working. The order often can be used to attach income from many other sources, including tax refund monies, pensions, unemployment checks, retirement benefits, etc. The order will also be in place when he gets another job.

Other avenues to explore when attempting to collect back–child support are federal and state income tax refunds and property liens. These are complicated methods, so you should consult an attorney to help you in these areas.

A court may also incarcerate the father for contempt of court if he refuses to make support payments. In some states, child support and child support enforcement is a civil matter. However, in others, it is a criminal offense for a father not to pay court ordered child support.

In some states, courts have developed child support enforcement procedures which can be used without the assistance of a lawyer. Court clerks can assist you in filling out and filing the appropriate forms.

Alternatively, consult with a private attorney, or get the criminal division of your local county or district attorneys office involved in the matter. The district attorneys office in the city in which you live can give you more information on this or any process concerning enforcement of a child support order.

Again, contact the Administration for Children and Families,

Office of Child Support Enforcement if you are having problems. Or, for $5.00, you can order an information kit on child support, child custody, and divorce from the NOW Legal Defense and Education Fund. Call (212)925–6635 to order a kit. For additional referrals, see the Resource Section at the end of this book.

Cracking down on "dead–beat" dads.

In 1989, uncollected child support was estimated to be in excess of $16 billion dollars. By 1995, that amount had grown 112%, to $34 billion. Unfortunately, state and county case workers are assigned 3,500 to 5,000 cases each, resulting in a bogged–down system that cannot realistically help all of those in need of assistance. Nonetheless, in recent years, most states are beginning to crack down on non–payment of child support.

In many states, laws have been enacted wherein licenses of various professionals, including licenses for teachers, lawyers, medical doctors can be suspended or revoked for non–payment. However, these are drastic measures which require several stages of non–payment of child support. In some states driver's licenses are not renewed if there are outstanding support payments due.

Private collection agencies.

There are also privately run organizations that will collect your back child support and spousal support. They operate in the same manner as a collection agency. Such organizations charge on a contingency (percentage) basis. Thus, if they do not collect any monies, clients should not be charged a fee.

Because the incentive and livelihood for these types of companies is based upon a percentage of the collected support, they are apt to pursue your support payments vigorously. Therefore, the results can be quicker and more effective than going through state or local agencies. One such national organization is Find Dad, Inc. To find out more about the services they provide, call (800)–PAY–MOMS.

Who gets the tax dependency exemption?

Invariably, both parents think they are entitled to the tax dependency exemption. But generally, absent any language or agreement to the contrary, the residential parent is the parent entitled to the IRS dependency exemption for the child.

In some cases, however, the dependency exemption can be negotiated or awarded to the paying parent. This may be within a court's discretion to decide. In some cases, the court will alternate the years for the exemption between the two parties if their relative incomes are essentially equal.

In the event of two children, the court will often give one tax exemption to each parent. Generally, the tax dependency exemption can only be used by the payor father if he is current in child support.

How long is my child's father obligated to make support payments?

Depending upon the laws of your state, support may continue past age 18 or until high school graduation, however, not past the age of 19, unless there is a physical or mental handicap requiring continuing support thereafter.

Some states may require a payment of schooling or college expenses for a child. But you will need to determine the exact laws of the state in which you reside.

VISITATION

If the natural father of your child decides to pursue his right to visitation, you should be aware that he has an absolute legal (if not moral) right to do so. The fact that you may not have been married to the father of your child is irrelevant in a court of law.

More and more, father's are opting for visitation rights.

Today we see that many more fathers are interested in participating in their children's lives. Very often they wish to enjoy activities and responsibilities that were once considered to be the mother's domain.

These days, more fathers are asking for, and demanding, these rights. Because of the changes in social expectations, the male parenting role is no longer such a passive one. You may find that although you and the father are not together as a couple, he may still chose to have a relationship with his child.

Hopefully you will understand and accept that your child needs his father. You may even encourage such a relationship, understanding that the benefits of a loving relationship between your child and his father is very important. Children are clearly best off when they have the advantage of both parents in their lives — providing they are both emotionally healthy, caring people.

It is better for your child to have to adjust to two different sets of household rules and family values than to do without his or her natural father. When your child's father is active in his or her life, you will also need to make adjustments.

When there is friction between a child's mother and father, emotions tend to run high, and ultimately the child pays the price. Often in these situations, people say and do things they later regret, and this causes the situation to get even worse. You may be sad, angry, or hurt. But it is important to work out your differences for the sake of your child. It is unfair and damaging to place him in the middle of an emotionally hostile or depressed environment.

If your child's father wishes to have visitation privileges with his child, it is far better emotionally, (as well as financially), to try and handle the issue constructively and fairly, rather than waging a war against one another and leaving it to the court to decide.

Visitation will require that you give up time with your child that you would prefer to spend with your child. Your focus, however, needs to be your child's best interests, and not necessarily your own. Most of the time, being a good parent means putting your child's needs first. Your child should be free to establish a good and healthy relationship with his father whenever possible.

It is also important for your child to see you getting along with her dad. She will learn about relationships from you. If your relationships have integrity, open communication, and mutual respect, these are the types of behavior she will adopt. Conversely, if you are angry, resentful, demanding, stubborn, hostile, or the like, she will reflect these attitudes in her own relationships.

Hopefully, you will never use your child as a pawn to get back at "him" for whatever you believe he may have done to you, and vice versa. Learn to conduct yourself with integrity and level headedness when dealing with your child's father.

An amicable resolution.

The absence or presence of the father in your child's life is going to bring different blessings, problems, and feelings for all of you — according to your circumstances. Whatever situations you must face, do your best to find the most amicable resolution to your differences, and meet your challenges with a positive attitude. This will go a long way to making everybody more happy.

Communication between you and your child's father will be your best means of resolving the issue of visitation between you. If you are having difficulty communicating with one another, counseling or attendance at various parenting courses may be beneficial for both of you.

If you are unable to resolve the issues between you, a court may have to step in to provide court–ordered provisions which both of you will need to abide by. However, if you can possibly avoid it, you really do not want to leave it up to the courts to decide your fate. The court's decision will likely leave one or both parties quite dissatisfied.

Visitation can be a joyful nurturing time for both parents and the child, or it can be a tedious, disruptive issue for all of you. Ultimately it depends on the attitudes taken.

Can my child's father visit with our child just because he pays child support?

Unless you agree otherwise, your child's father can not see your child until he gets a court order to do so. The duty to pay child support and the right to visit your child are two different things. In the eyes of the law, they are not connected.

My child's father is seeking visitation through the courts. What can I expect will happen?

In such a case, it is very likely that the father will prevail and the court will order visitation. In fact, courts presume that it is healthy and important for a child to have a relationship with *both* parents. These days, many courts are ordering "shared parental responsibility" as opposed to "sole parental responsibility". This means that *both* parents are *equal* parents in the eyes of the law.

These rights include access and visitation to the child no matter which parent provides the custody or primary residence to the child. Furthermore, major decisions affecting the life of the child should be discussed and agreed upon in a co–parenting fashion considering the best interests of the child.

Unfortunately, this is not always easy because one parent is the custodial parent and is more involved in the child's every–day life. And in some instances, the parents may not get along with one another or share the same beliefs or values. Nonetheless, when shared parental responsibility is ordered, the non–custodial parent is entitled to school records, medical records, participation in activities of the child, attendance at teacher conferences, and involvement in all other aspects of the child's life unless such involvement can be proven to be detrimental.

Courts are loathe to restrict a parent's right to a child. However, if a parent (in this case the father) is shown to be potentially detrimental to your child (i.e., he is abusive, or a child molester, etc.), a court may restrict his access or say–so with regard to your child. In this case, the court's may require supervised visitation, restrict overnight visitation, or require counseling of one or both parents. Be advised, however, when parents try to restrict or prevent access to a child by the other parent for no good cause, the courts generally deem such behavior to be harmful to the child and look down upon it.

Ultimately, visitation and custody issues are within a court's absolute discretion and power to decide. The court will make a determinations based upon what is in the child's best interest, not what the parents prefer. It does not matter whether you like or respect your child's father, or that do not want him to see your child. A court will consider such feelings to be irrelevant or even hold such feelings against you to your detriment.

Visitation guidelines.

Although visitation is determined on a case by case basis, many jurisdictions have minimal guidelines for visitation. These guidelines may include visitation every other weekend from Friday until Sunday, one–half of holidays, 2–12 weeks during each summer and possibly other time during each week.

The visitation may also include provisions for Father's Day, Mother's Day, both parties' birthdays, the child's birthday, teacher holidays, work schedules, and three–day weekends. The courts might also determine specified times and locations of pick–up and drop–off; who has the responsibility of pick–up and drop–off; shared driving arrangements, etc.

The court may also assign cost in visitation to the other party in cases of long distance visitation. However, the variations of circumstances must be reviewed on a case by case basis, because while for some, visitation may work out great with liberal language included in the visitation order, others may need their lives ordered to the very minute.

My child is confused by two sets of rules in two separate households. How do I deal with this issue?

If your child visits with her father in his home, you may find that there are some conflicts between the two of you with respect to the subject of discipline, expectations, house rules, etc. Dad may have one set of rules for his house and you may have another for yours. Good communication between you and dad with respect to your differences is therefore important.

Try to be flexible with him, and he will more likely to be flexible with you. Of course, sometimes, when two people completely disagree, no amount of communication will bridge the gap.

Stephanie, a divorced mother I know, insists that her son wear socks with his shoes. To her, this is important — yet her ex could care less about socks. Of course, his values regarding this issue are equally as important to him as Stephanie's are to her.

Oftentimes, when Stephanie's son returns home, he has no socks on his feet which infuriates Stephanie. For her, socks on her child's feet are a important. But instead of being flexible, she gets "into it" with her child's father. Pretty soon, the kid is a mess, she's angry and Dad accuses her of being a nag.

The moral here is this: If you and your child's father cannot agree on certain issue, unless it harms your child, and you are willing to go to war over it, let dad do what he does in his home and you follow the rules in your house.

You will want to communicate to your child when she is old enough that *"Daddy has certain rules in his house, and Mommy has certain rules in hers, and they are not always the same rules. I know it's hard to have two sets of rules, but I expect you to follow the rules I set in our house."*

This may not entirely eliminate the conflict for your child, but open communication about this issue will help.

The fact is, conflicts concerning discipline, behaviors, house rules, etc., as between you and your child's father will not always be easy to deal with. Hopefully you can work them out by remaining calm, reasonable and flexible with one another.

CUSTODY

The mother *or* the father may get custody through the courts.

Where the issue of custody is concerned, the courts may not discriminate against one parent or the other on the basis of gender. In fact, many courts have abolished the "tender years doctrine" wherein the court would give preference and consider as a factor the young age of the child in awarding custody to the mother. The fact that you may not have been married to the baby's father is also irrelevant. A court will grant custody based on what it believes is in the child's best interests.

While historically courts have granted physical custody to the mother, mother bias has begun to change in recent years. Although judges may still show certain trends toward a mother versus a father, many judges are neutral and consider all factors. And thus, more and more, we see fathers asking for and getting custody or shared custody; and most states have adopted rules allowing shared custody to take place. These days, anything can happen.

When custody is a contested issue, it is recommended that a parent not step near a courtroom without a family law attorney. The reality is that the high stakes in a custody battle will determine a child's entire future. And if a mother loses custody, she may be required to pay child support to the father.

Child support can go both ways. Moreover, upon loss of a child custody suit, the losing parent will then receive the much higher burden of showing a change of circumstances for a modification of custody in the future.

If your child's father can prove that you are an unfit parent, or demonstrate to the court that the child's best interests would be served by living with him, it is possible that the court could choose to award custody to him.

To decide the issue of custody, the courts will look carefully at both parents lifestyles, work responsibilities, ability to care for the children, etc.

Joint physical custody.

Many court jurisdictions frown upon "joint physical custody". Joint physical custody, where a child lives with both parents on a split–basis, is often considered to be detrimental and is presumed to create upheaval and instability in a child's life. Judges may even throw out such an arrangement made between the parents if they do not consider it to be in the child's best interest.

Nevertheless, with the proper psychological evaluation stating there will be no ill effect, and in consideration of the child's age, courts may accept such an arrangement. However, they are not commonplace. You should consult with an attorney to find out more about joint physical custody in your jurisdiction.

Using a custody battle to intimidate.

It is a sad reality that children are often used to hurt, intimidate or cause trouble for the other parent; and a custody battle is a powerful way to accomplish this. There are also times when children are "used" without a parent's conscious recognition that this is what they are doing.

Whatever the motivation, the act of using a child in this way is a totally selfish, self–centered and destructive thing to do. It is important when discussing the issue of child custody to ask ourselves "What is in the best interest of my child and, am I being selfish in pressing my claim?"

Regretfully, visitation or custody battles are one of the pitfalls of split homes — and sometimes we must deal with it whether we like it or not. If, after you have exhausted all other avenues, you must go to court to resolve these issues, here are some guidelines for you to follow (some of these ideas will also help you strengthen your overall parenting skills):

- Attempt to be cordial (and friendly if possible) with your child's father. You should be aware that anything you say, do or write to him can and may be used against you at a future date to prove to a court that you are an unfit parent. Keep in mind that your child will be affected by any negative relationship you have with her father.
- Take good care of your children! Make sure that they are well fed, have clean clothes, are appropriately groomed, attend school regularly, and have lots of love! You do not want the court to see you as an unsuitable custodial parent.
- Do not bad–mouth your child's father in front of your child. A court will not look favorably upon this and it is extremely hurtful to your child.
- Show your willingness to make compromises by attending mediation, counseling, arbitration, or other alternatives to fighting it out. A court is likely to look more favorably upon a parent willing to resolve conflicts peacefully.
- Do not use your children as a go–between, messenger, or spy.
- Do not use your child to get back at "him" for those things you perceive he did wrong to you.
- Put any and all oral agreements between you and your child's father in writing, sign the document and submit it to the court for a court order.
- Your willingness to have a positive relationship with the father should help you in a custody battle and is always better for

your child.

PARENTING – DOING IT ON YOUR OWN

Parenting is a wonderful adventure full of challenges and surprises. The depth of the joy, love, tenderness — and even the sadness and frustration we experience — is a gift and blessing to our lives. You are remarkable in your courage, strength and determination to give your child a good life even when the odds — and prevailing negative opinions of our culture — are against you.

You may have a tough road to travel. And you will need to overcome many challenges — without the aid of a loving partner to help you through it. But your own strength, courage and determination will go a long way toward lighting your path and bringing you the answers you need when the questions arise.

I hope that you will set an example for those around you who have negative views about single–parenting. Through your courage, tenacity, resourcefulness and creativity, you can show them that a single–parent can indeed make a family whole. You can raise your child with the love, security and devotion it is generally believed only comes through a two-parent family.

There will be times when all is well in your life and the life of your child or children. There will be other times when you will wonder: "How can I get through this?" With all of it's inherent difficulties, the answer is really simple. In difficult times, you put one foot in front of the other and walk through the circumstances, certain that you will get to the other side. In the end, our children make it all worth while.

IN CONCLUSION

Both individually and as a society, it is time to do some work to make a more substantial investment in our childrens' futures. Because the problems our children face are problems for all of society, it is imperative that we take positive, pro–active steps to ensure that our children receive all of the advantages we can possibly provide. *It is time to focus on the well–being of our children because they are the future.*

—*CHAPTER FOURTEEN*—

MY STORY

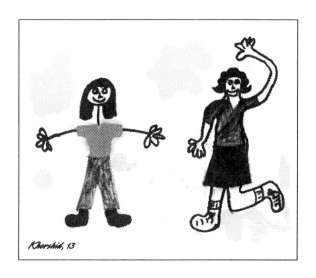

Khorshid, 13

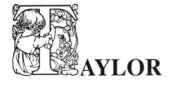

AYLOR

During my first pregnancy, I was calm, joyous, and coolheaded. Overall, my temperament — hormonally speaking — was fairly predictable. I felt terrific. I was fortunate enough not to have any morning sickness or serious mood swings. I basically floated through the experience, finding it to be a delightful and wondrous adventure — notwithstanding the fact that I was determined to "do it" alone, without a husband.

My son's father and I were casually involved for a rather brief period of time. When we started out, there was no relationship on the horizon for us, let alone a baby. I did not love this man, and he did not love me.

When I unexpectedly found myself pregnant, I was genuinely surprised. But I was comfortable with the idea of becoming a single mother. The decision to have this child was solely my choice from the first moment. So, despite the fact that Taylor's father and I had no intention of being together, I still desired and longed to have this child and knew that somehow he was meant to be born to me.

Several years earlier, I had been married to a terrific man who died after we'd been together only seven years. Needless to say, I was crushed when he died, and mistakenly believed that I would not find love again in my lifetime. The baby growing within me felt like an opportunity to learn to love again — and to be loved.

At the time I became pregnant, I was feeling emotionally, spiritually, chronologically (I was 28 years old) ready and eager for this child. Since my husband had died, I had been doing a lot of serious work to heal myself and to become vibrantly alive again. Additionally, I had a very good job and was for the most part, financially secure. I was sure I could handle all of the obligations, challenges and responsibilities of being a single–parent.

I wasn't particularly frightened about having a baby without a partner. I was excited — especially since all of my good friends supported me with their belief in my ability to "do it" by myself.

There were, of course, other, more casual acquaintances — and even people whom I did not know well at all — who were more pessimistic and discouraging toward the situation. Those were the voices of doubt and fear, doom and gloom. They emphasized the difficulties and drawbacks of having a child on my own, and warned me not to do it.

Fortunately for me, those voices were in the minority and I paid no attention to them. Instead, I listened to my heart and to the people who knew and loved me best. So, that was it. Once and for all I decided I was going to have a baby by myself without the assistance of my baby's biological father.

I was thrilled with my decision to have this baby. Yes it would be difficult, but I would take on the challenge like "The Little Train That Could" saying to myself "I know I can...I know I can". And so I did.

Looking back, I'd have to say that my attitude was what made the experience so delightfully wonderful for me. I knew it wouldn't always be a piece of cake, for I was looking at the world of motherhood and babies realistically, not through rose colored glasses.

I understood the challenges and difficulties of babies and accepted that my life would change. I knew I would have to sacrifice certain of the liberties and freedoms that I had become accustomed to as a young single woman responsible only for myself. But I was ready! I made a mental decision to see my son as an addition to my life, and not as a detraction from it.

My son was born on Christmas eve, 1988. What a magnificent dream it was which had come to life before my very eyes! No one could have told me what the experience of becoming a mother would be like.

Although labor and delivery were lengthy and difficult, this child seemed to me to be the most perfect baby ever born. He was so beautiful (every mother's baby is), and he was my new family.

The moment I looked at Taylor, I knew that my life had changed forever and that I would do anything for him. Still, it took me a good while to really fall "in love" with him, at least longer than "they" say in baby books. I suppose I was afraid that if I gave myself to him emotionally, or accepted him too deeply within my heart that, like my deceased husband, he, too, would leave me. A ridiculous notion I fear, but emotions are not level–headed.

After I left the hospital, I remember walking through the front door of my small, one bedroom apartment, with my new baby in my arms and a rush of shock came over me. No nurses, doctors, friends — no anybody there but me and this baby. It was such a strange feeling. I felt isolated and a little afraid. I didn't know what I was supposed to do with him — and I don't mean for the next week, month, year, or rest of his life. I didn't know what to do with him in the very next moment; and the moment after that.

The idea came to me that we had to have a talk. And so I began to babble to this small, brand new baby. I must have looked pretty silly telling this newborn infant about the "house rules".

I explained to Taylor that I was new at this; that I wasn't sure what I was supposed to do, and that we had better come to some basic understandings. If he would be accommodating to me, I would be accommodating to him. No major crying bouts (a small amount to let me know he was hungry was okay), regular sleeping hours would be nice; and he had to go with me wherever I went and be charming to all the nice people we would meet.

The funny thing is, it seemed as if he understood me. Taylor was generally a very peaceful, quiet baby with little crying, no colic, and no diaper rashes. He was independent and would often entertain himself for hours at a time with the same toy. As far as I could tell, we were off to a very good start. For the first few months, it seemed as if I was beginning to get this motherhood thing under control — and for the most part, was doing it with relative ease and little discomfort.

I was especially fortunate when the answer to my initial child care dilemma was overcome. My boss, who was very kind and understanding toward me and my situation, allowed me to bring my son to the law office where I worked. Taylor was so amazingly quiet, cheerful, and calm that I was able to handle him easily — with a little help from the office staff.

After Taylor had been coming to the office for about three or four months, however, others began to notice that he was less active than most babies his age — that he was very much like a rag doll in terms of his muscle control. They also commented on his passive nature (I thought I just got a "good" baby).

At that point in time, as I struggled with the typical dilemmas of parenting — and those that go along with single–parenting, it was becoming clear that certain things about Taylor were unusual. I began to understand that there were greater problems for us to face together.

When Taylor was 10 months old, he could not hold his head up and would slip through one's hands if he wasn't held closely. He didn't have the reflexes or muscle control to automatically flex and tighten up his muscles as was normal for babies his age. At 10 months, Taylor could neither roll over, nor get up on his knees to crawl.

Finally, my doctor suggested that I take Taylor to a neurologist for tests. I went to a specialist who was recommended to me by my doctor and remember sitting in his office after his examination with fear in my heart and panic in my brain. What was he going to tell me about my baby?

Taylor was diagnosed with global "hypotonia" and global developmental delays. Essentially both of these problems had to do with his ability to do such things as hold his head up, crawl, walk, etc., at the average age when most babies would do them. I was told that at his age, all I could do was to wait and see what developed. I was told that his situation was borderline and that only time would indicate the extent of the "problem". I was told that often these "problems" straighten themselves out and that some babies are just delayed in these areas.

Initially, I was devastated over Taylor's situation. How could this happen? It took me several months to adjust to our circumstance, to accept the situation as it was, to stop asking "why?", and to allow it to unfold on its own.

I began to see that I also had the choice to determine how I was going to experience this "problem". So I decided at once to have a more positive attitude about it — though this was a big step for me. I stopped calling Taylor's situation a "problem" because I felt that doing so kept me in a negative place. Instead, I began to refer to it as our "situation". This really helped a lot to eliminate much of the negativity I was experiencing.

Since I could not alter the situation, and no medical help was possible at this early age, I had to deal with my own reaction — and that wasn't always easy. But I knew I needed to resolve my feelings about the circumstances which were mine. I had to find a way to get through and over my son's limitations.

It was at about this point when I learned one of the greatest lessons I have ever received. Looking closely at my circumstances and my reaction to it, I was able to see that I was placing conditions upon my son. I wanted everything to be perfect. I wanted him to be perfect. Who doesn't? What I finally came to see, however, was that with all of its imperfections, the situation — and my child — were indeed perfect — exactly as they were.

As Taylor grew, he would ultimately overcome one obstacle (or delay) only to encounter another. It was a cycle I came to know well. Taylor's delays were a challenge for both of us, and at times frustrating to the point of tears. But I continued to look for answers.

When Taylor was about 1-1/2 years old, I was told by a neurologist that Taylor might never walk. That was a hard pill to swallow. It took a lot of soul searching to come to terms with that possibility. But I came to feel that whether he walked or not, he was my perfect baby and I loved him so much more than I could have imagined before he came into my life.

Around that same time, I had the added challenge of incurring overwhelming financial responsibilities and obligations. With the cost of the doctors added to the cost of raising a child, among other unexpected incidents in my life, I needed help. In fact, circumstances were so bad that I could no longer ignore the idea that Taylor's father had an obligation to assist his son.

I had been putting off going to court to seek child support. Finally, with the help of friends who pointed out to me that it was not about my pride, but about Taylor's needs, I saw it was the right thing for me to do. When Taylor was nearly two years old I engaged an attorney to assist me to collect child support.

I tried to work out something with Taylor's father first. But he told me that his "side of the street was clean" and that this was my "karma". Ultimately, the court's did not agree.

Much to my delight, around Taylor's second birthday, one day, out of the blue, he got up and took his first steps. I was not there to see it happen. I was at work and he was with his babysitter. When I found out, I cried and cried, as most mothers do when their child does such things for the first time. More than that milestone though, was the relief that my son would walk.

The first time I got to see Taylor walk was a few days later. He had been practicing for me. He was my miracle unfolding right there in front of my eyes. Still, we were to have numerous challenges ahead of us.

On the child support front, after a rather lengthy period of dealing with lawyers and the court, the court finally ordered Taylor's father to pay child support (a rather small amount) beginning when Taylor was approximately three years old.

Taylor's father made regular, somewhat timely payments for several months. Generally the check, which was due on the first of the month, would arrive by the fifteenth; and the check for the fifteenth would arrive around the first of the next month. As time passed, however, the time in between the payments began to grow longer until finally the payments just stopped coming altogether.

When Taylor's father ignored my requests to get back on track with the payments, I decided to take control of the matter. I had delayed taking more serious action toward collecting the long–overdue support because I was still hoping he'd do the right thing. But after about a year when it became clear that he wasn't going to do the right thing, I contacted the District Attorneys Office in my area. I involved the D.A.'s office in collecting the over due child support payments because it seemed illogical to me to pay high attorneys fees in order to collect court–ordered money we needed.

The District Attorney's office had the case (probably collecting dust) for over a year. After getting tired of waiting for them to take action, I wrote letters demanding that they handle the case and not just continue to brush me off.

After several more weeks with no response, I obtained the personal fax number of the District Attorney (the real man behind the title). I then faxed the letter to him each and every morning when I got into work, with a stamp marked "Still waiting for your reply" stamped over and over, dated each and every day I sent it. Within a few weeks, I received a letter indicating that they had turned the case over to the prosecution division for some serious action.

Thankfully, the prosecution division took a shorter period of time to resolve the issue. They had the file for only three months before an agreement was made between Taylor's father and the D.A.'s office resolving the issue of back–support and continuing support.

Taylor was 6 years old when his father was again ordered to make child support payments, but this time he was put on probation with the understanding that if he missed more than three months worth of payments at a time, the D.A. would reopen the file and prosecute him.

The whole ordeal was draining and annoying. But mostly, I was surprised to see first–hand the lack of integrity one man can have toward himself and his child. Though he may not have "wanted" this child, it did not not relieve him of any moral or legal obligation to care for him financially. Of course, he continus to blame me, thinks I'm terrible, and speaks unkindly about me. I don't know why I ever expected more of him.

In the beginning, Taylor's father spent time with him, taking him for weekends or short visits. But eventually he stopped seeing Taylor altogether, though occasionally we do run into him. On those infrequent occasions, he treats Taylor as if he were someone else's child. It is very sad for both of them, especially Taylor. And it hurts me immensely to see my son trying to figure out why his daddy doesn't care for him.

Overall, Taylor appears to handle the situation very well. We talk openly about his father when he brings him up. I presume more of his feelings will surface as he gets older. But for now, we cope with it the best we can.

With respect to my son's developmental delays, today Taylor walks, runs, and speaks. But there is one catch: Taylor is autistic. He was diagnosed with "high functioning autism" in May, 1995. He was, by then, 6 years old.

When the specialist at UCLA told me that Taylor was autistic, I was numb. I was partly relieved (I had searched for years to find out what made Taylor "different" from other kids his age), and was partly devastated.

Autism is a spectrum disorder. Each individual who has the dis-order is different from the next. I have come to find that autism is very misunderstood — and "high functioning" is often subjective. People think of "Rain Man" but that's not how my child is.

I would describe my son as special, and in some ways, eccen-tric. One day he appears to be perfectly "normal" or "typical" — and the next he seems "different" than his peers.

There exists in my life a constant battle with the school system, teachers, state–run agencies who provide programs for Taylor, and others. But the battles have been worth it. My (many) battles to obtain services, and early intervention for Taylor have, without a doubt, created the opportunity for Taylor to excel and overcome many difficulties.

Today, after several years of special education classes, Taylor is fully–included in a regular classroom. He is, academically speaking, highly gifted, talented, friendly, smiles a lot, and loves even more.

Taylor's autism has reminded me that we don't always get to be in control of life. That's just the way it is. Our children will be and do certain things that we have no ability to change. Life may hand us cards that we can't make sense of. What we must do is work with the things we can change and learn to accept the rest with grace.

Coming to this conclusion early on turned out to be a perfect opportunity for me to learn about acceptance. It might otherwise have taken me a lifetime to learn this important lesson had I not had this experience to help me grow as a person and as a mother.

Through this experience, I have learned to savor my blessings and accept my challenges. I have chosen to try to look at life's curve balls as opportunities for growth. And more often than not, I succeed.

FINDING LOVE AGAIN

When Taylor was eleven months old, I met a man named Danny. We became involved in a long–term, on–and–off again relationship.

At first, the relationship was against my better judgment, because in truth, I wasn't prepared to fall in love. I was contented to date and have a good time – no attachments, no commitments, or so I thought.

As the days and weeks passed, Danny continued to pursue me and I was flattered. Then one day, I woke up to discover that I had fallen in love with this wonderful man. I adored him and considered him to be my best friend — and the love of my life. And so the dance began.

ꓙACE: *Pregnant Again.*

I was so happy the day I found out I was pregnant with my second baby. I was also miserable. Those two emotions rolled into one confirmed in my mind that I was, quite frankly, a basket case. I wasn't sure that I wanted to have another child. Taylor was nearly six years old, I was busy with my full time job, a side business, commitments in various organizations I belonged to, a social life, and Danny and his three kids. Was I ready to have another baby? Well, at least this time my baby would have a daddy — or so I thought.

I had suspected for a few weeks that I was pregnant, but I didn't say a word to Danny. I wanted to make sure before I talked to him about it. When the purple line on the home pregnancy test came out blaring "You're pregnant!" I was silently happy about it but outwardly afraid. I instantly fell in love with this child because I loved Danny so much and this baby was a part of both of us. I was so sure that Danny would look upon this "happy" event as a miracle as well; a blessing; a welcome addition to our lives.

About a year before, I had a false alarm, thinking that I might be pregnant. When I got my period and told Danny "Good news, I'm not pregnant" he was silent. I asked if he was okay because he didn't sound very happy about it over the telephone. He told me that he was a little disappointed —that he was kind of looking forward to having a baby with me. I guess I subconsciously filed this information away for future reference.

Our relationship over the years had been a love affair with the best and the worst of each other. I fell in love with his children and he with my son. And though we never lived together, in an odd way, we were a family. And yet we were far from ever really being a family in the traditional sense. Still, I loved the little "family" we had created.

Over the years, Danny and I gave and took so much from one another, yet in the end, it seemed that all we held on to was resentment and pain. And though we loved each other very much, as long as we were holding on to our pain it couldn't be enough to make the relationship work.

Mostly, from my perspective, it was a "timing thing". When I wanted more of a commitment, Danny didn't. When he was ready and wanted to marry me, I wasn't emotionally available to him. We were, as I often called us, "windshield wipers in time" — never really together, and never really apart.

Ultimately, I guess our back and forth relationship, and the mixed messages we gave to one another, built up such deep resentments that we both took them out on one another in our own destructive ways. The sad thing was that though we really loved each other, we just couldn't find a way to give up the old anger and work things out — at least not at the same time. Of course, he blamed me, and I blamed him. The truth is, we were both responsible for our own part in the whole mess.

That Friday afternoon after I took the home pregnancy test, Danny came to pick me up. We were going to spend our usual weekend together at his house, with all the kids. I had been sick over the preceding few days and was taking antibiotics. He asked me if I remembered to bring them with me. I was silent for a few moments and stared at him, puzzled and unsure of what to say. I wasn't sure that I should be taking any medication now, knowing that I was pregnant.

Danny looked at me in that strange way that he often did when it seemed he was reading my mind. He asked "Are you pregnant?" I just blurted it out. Yes I was. It wasn't exactly the way I wanted to tell him. Not very sensitive or tactful, but there it was. It had come out.

I smiled and tried to crack a joke to lighten the shocked look on his face. He was stunned, but I didn't know how stunned until later. We rode in silence to the market where we had planned to go to get some things for the weekend. In the market, he leaned over to me and asked if my insurance covered pregnancy. Unfortunately it didn't. Still, his question gave me some hope that he was considering this to be an okay thing — that he was going to accept it after all.

We spent the weekend in an awkward silence. At one point on Saturday morning at breakfast, Taylor announced to the kids "Me and Mommy are going to have a baby." Danny's kids laughed and thought he was just kidding. Yea I thought to myself, "just kidding".

Finally, by Sunday morning the tension was so great that Danny drove me home. I don't even remember how we came to agree that I would go home. I just know that suddenly I was in the car and we were at a loss to say much of anything. I thought to myself: "Well, he's still just in shock, he doesn't know what to say or do."

At the time, Danny and I worked in the same office. On the following Monday morning, I came in to the office and sitting on my computer was an overstuffed envelope with Danny's handwriting adorning the front of it. My heart sank. What was in the letter that he couldn't say to me face to face?

I knew the contents before I even read the letter. I sat down cautiously and began to read Danny's words: He "...did not want this baby", it was a "mistake", and our problems were so great he didn't know if "we'd be together through the summer let alone the child's youth.", etc., etc.

Five pages of Danny, and nothing about me or my feelings. He didn't ask how was I feeling; didn't ask what I wanted to do, and didn't seem to want to know how afraid I was. After five years together, it all seemed to come down to how this was going to ruin his life. I was devastated. I felt so alone; so very alone.

The next day, I took a leave of absence from my job to take two weeks to figure out what I was going to do. I couldn't bear to see Danny's face at the office every day while I was trying to hold it all together. So I went off to New York over the Fourth of July weekend to see my sister. I tried to have a good time, and almost succeeded; but I wasn't fooling anyone, least of all myself.

While I was in New York, I must have seen at least ten of those pro–life commercials with those oh–so–adorable kids doing those oh–so–adorable things while the narrator says something like "These kids weren't planned, but oh look at them now!" Charming. I was mildly toying with the idea that I should just go and have an abortion. End this whole mess. How could I possibly have a baby alone – – again? But those commercials really got to me.

I'm not personally against abortion. I believe in a woman's right to choose. Every woman has different limitations, abilities, and emotional responses. But for me, in my heart of hearts, having an abortion was not what I wanted to do. Under the circumstances however, I was considering the idea. I just wanted the terrible emotional pain to go away.

The idea of having a child alone, again, was initially heart–wrenching. I had always said that doing it alone once was fine but twice was crazy. I wanted to be married and in love if and when I conceived another child. A second single pregnancy was not what I had in mind.

New York and two weeks away from the office, were helpful. But they weren't enough to clear the fog from my head or remove the crazy ideas and thoughts that were going through my mind.

During this time, I didn't go to the doctor but calculated that I was approximately 7 weeks pregnant. I couldn't even get an abortion until I was 8 weeks along so I still had a little bit of time. Even with all the confusion and upset, my heart resisted the notion of terminating my pregnancy while my mind created all kinds of negative scenarios. I felt as if I was suffocating.

I was depressed and lonely, and so I began to visit my church Wednesday evenings in addition to my usual attendance on Sunday mornings. I consider myself to be more spiritual than religious. Fortunately, my church is unconditionally loving and does not judge me as a "sinner" for becoming pregnant out of wedlock.

My church family was there to support me. The time I spent in church seemed to be the only time I was able to be at peace in my heart and mind, and it was there that I came to know what I needed to do.

MAKING THE DECISION TO KEEP MY BABY

I am fortunate enough to have two mothers in my life (it's a long story). However, my natural mother did not support my decision to have my baby. Thankfully, my adoptive mother did. She helped me to see that I could do this and encouraged me every step of the way. When I had moments of doubt, she reassured me that everything would be alright — and somehow I believed her.

Throughout those months of difficulty, while I struggled to find my way, it was an even harder time for Taylor. He had lost his "daddy" and was very confused. He loved Danny so much and suddenly he was gone from our lives.

It was so hard not to be self–obsessed and become lifeless when I got home from work and on weekends. At times it was even harder to be strong for Taylor. It would have been easy to stay in bed and isolate. I worked at keeping busy and resisted the inclination to feel sorry for myself. I made plans to go out and do things with friends. I went for morning walks, and evening swims. And I engaged in activities with Taylor to keep us both going.

At this point, things at the office were getting out of hand. Danny was doing everything he could to get me to have an abortion. And he was reaching new levels of low behavior. I felt manipulated, coerced, and abandoned. I kept praying that he would wake up and see how unkindly he was treating me.

At one point it seemed as though my prayers had been answered. Danny began to be nice to me again. I was so astonished and happy. I was full of hope that he really did love me after all and that he would come around. We had a few dinners and one evening I stayed over at his house. But that night when we went to sleep, something was missing. Danny almost always held me very closely when we slept together. But this night he couldn't even put his arms around me. I suspect he couldn't bring himself to touch my stomach which was beginning to expand.

I felt as if Danny hated me and the baby I was carrying. I was silently crushed, but didn't share that with him. I didn't dare rock the boat and ask him about it. I tried so hard to be loving and supportive of his feelings. I even tried not to talk about the baby — fearing it would set him off. But eventually I became very bitter and resentful toward him.

Finally, one Monday evening the boundaries between us were clearly drawn. We had a confrontation, and I got in my car to drive home. On the way, I found myself saying over and over to myself "I can't do this, I just can't do this!". When I got home I called Danny to tell him he'd "won", to have a check to me by Friday, and that I'd make an appointment for an abortion. I hung up the phone before he could respond. Two days later he put a check for the abortion on my desk.

On Tuesday morning, I made an appointment to have an abortion the following Friday. But over the next several days, I began to sink to a new emotional low. At one point I thought to myself "If I stop drinking water and eating, how long will it take for me to die?" I felt despondent and depressed and wasn't sure how I could possibly pull myself out of it.

I was so afraid of my feelings that I decided I needed to see a therapist to help me overcome the negative thoughts I was having. I scheduled a meeting with a new therapist on Wednesday — two days before my appointment to have an abortion. At our first session, I spent the whole hour crying and sharing my sadness and pain over the rejection I felt from my mother and from Danny.

Then the therapist gave me an assignment — which helped me to have a great shift in my attitude. She asked that I write 100 times, the affirmation she created for me: "I am a beautiful woman, physically and in my soul." In the right–hand corner, after each sentence, I was to write the first thought that came to my mind.

At first, the right column looked like a pitiful, negative flow of words. But as I continued to write, the left column began to hold some possibilities: "I can try to believe this", "I need to work for this", "maybe".

It was rather strange, but about two hours after I had finished the assignment, I began to feel some hope. Maybe I really was a "beautiful woman, physically and in my soul!" I began to hear the laughter from the other workers in the office not as an annoyance, as I had for so many weeks, but as hope that I, too, could be laughing soon.

I canceled my appointment for Friday's intended abortion and instead made an appointment to see an obstetrician. I was going to keep my baby, and do it alone. On Thursday, I tore up the check, and I told Danny I would be having my child. He retorted angrily: "Just do what you're going to do."

The following Monday morning, I found another of his many letters on my desk. It read in part that "Lest there be any doubt...you may not have been fully listening or paying attention...I am through with you... stay away, stay away, stay away..." He told me that he would go "kicking and screaming into court" if I forced him, and that he would "use Taylor's father as an example of tieing me up in the court system. And Danny, an attorney himself, was fully capable of keeping me in court for a long time.

Danny went on to accuse me of getting pregnant on "purpose" (why do men do this — as if they weren't there, or at the very least accountable for their actions?) But I knew the truth and was determined to follow my heart.

The following Thursday, I went to see my doctor. When during the examination, the doctor turned to me and said "That's your baby's heartbeat", I was astonished. There it was this loud, swishing, thump, thump, thump. I was so overwhelmed by the rhythmic sound of this life, which only days before I had contemplated aborting, that tears rolled down my cheeks. These tears were happy, good tears.

That moment was the first moment in so many days and weeks that I felt peaceful and secure. I was still sad and hurt that Danny was not interested in being a part of this miracle — his child — and of my life with Taylor. But I knew with certainty in that instant that I had made the right decision to keep my child.

As my own inner strength began to improve and grow, I continued to pray that Danny would "let go of his anger", and find peace in his heart. I also prayed for my own peace and acceptance of the circumstances as they were — not as I would have them be.

Then one morning, a few weeks later, I found a card on my chair stuffed in some old lizard cowboy boots that Danny had returned to me. By this time I was leery of anything with his handwriting on it. Everything I had received to this point had been hurtful and angry. I took a deep breath, not wanting to open it and be hurt again. But instead of angry words, the card simply said "I've decided to let go of my anger".

There was no way to change the past, and the future was not holding any promises for us to be together. But at least the anger was less intense. I realized that I had no choice but to let go and accept the fact that I was going to be a single mother one more time.

I continued to do the same things to get me through the remainder of my pregnancy that I've since written about in this book. They began to take on a new meaning and real urgency for me. I began to do affirmations, physical exercise, meditation, prayer, therapy, etc. Anything that I could think of to help me through the combination of a broken heart, morning sickness, and hormonal craziness.

I also began to write my story. I discovered that writing was the best way to relieve some of the vast emptiness I was feeling. Expressing myself on paper provided a wonderful, necessary release.

I did not start out with the intention of writing a book. But as I wrote, I began to experience a catharsis which seemed to erase much of the doubt, worry, and fear that had engulfed me like a flame. When I took a pen in hand, it seemed as if the words just wrote themselves. I knew then that I had something important to say.

The process of writing became essential to my well–being during that pregnancy, and ultimately, my own words gave me much of the courage I needed to get through the rest of my pregnancy. They reminded me of what I needed to do, and how to create the experience I wanted.

One day as I was writing, I noticed a great shift in my feelings. A change in my perception and a new hope loomed in my heart. The idea to write this book came to me as a way to share my experience and reach out to others in a similar situation.

The choice to have a baby without a partner again held many mixed emotions, many challenges and many possibilities, and I was beginning to see them more for the better than for the worse. I began to remember and feel the same hope I had held in my heart and mind when I was pregnant with Taylor. To once again see the possibilities I had forgotten, and to allow more love to enrich my life, was now an exciting opportunity and possibility.

Out of love, I was bringing a baby into this world, and I was sure it was the right decision for me. The experience I had gained the first time around as a single–parent helped to quiet my concerns and fears. I began to hear and listen to my inner voice which told me over and over that my decision to have another baby was the right one.

As time went on, I began to feel stronger and more alive every day. The reality that a new baby boy would be joining Taylor and me as part of our family was very exciting. Taylor also enjoyed talking about "baby Jace", and being a part of the experience. We drew pictures together of the baby in mommy's tummy, and we talked about what it would be like when baby Jace came to live with us. Taylor looked forward to being my little helper.

In the end, my mother finally came around and was at the hospital when Jace was born. Danny also chose to be present at his son's birth and he has since continued to be there for his child. In fact, he loves both of his little boys so much. His presence is consistent in both of their lives, and he's turned out to be the best daddy any two little boys could have. Danny loves Taylor as his own son, and Jace is loved by him as much as any child could be.

I love both of my little boys so much. Each day I thank god for their grace and presence in my life. Today, when I see the light in Danny's eyes as he looks at Jace, I get teary–eyed to think of what I went through to have him — and then again, sometimes — I just smile. It was worth every moment of darkness to see this light. Jace has changed all of our lives forever.

In the end, I believe that everything in life happens for a reason — and nothing, but nothing — happens by accident. Ultimately, where one door closes, another one is waiting to be opened — and thus, this chapter cannot really be completed.

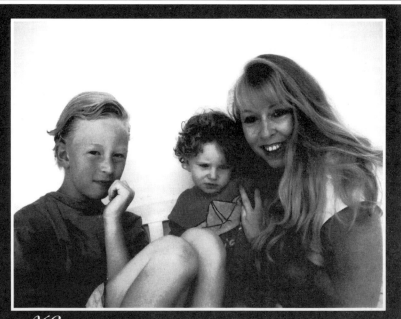

$\mathscr{K}$eri Bowers lives with her two sons, Taylor, 7-1/2, and Jace, 15 months, in Southern California. She is currently working on her next two books: "Molestation From a Child's Eyes" (in collaboration with two young girls, victims of sexual abuse); and "the Big Tiny Moon, Dispelling the Myths of High Funchioning Autism." Keri is also a motivational speaker on the topics of positive parenting; single parenting; and substance abuse.

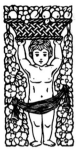

RESOURCES
SUPPORT GROUPS AND SERVICES

FAMILY RESOURCE COALITION
200 South Michigan Avenue, Suite 1600
Chicago, Illinois 60604
(312) 341–0900 fax (312) 341–9361

This organization is a membership, consulting, and advocacy organization whose goal is to strengthen and support families. For $5.00, you can purchase a guide for parents on starting and operating your own support group. It also offers other publications on a variety of topics including child care, prevention of child abuse, teen parents, welfare reform, and resources for African American and Latino families, among many others

LA LECHE LEAGUE
1400 North Meacham Road
Schaumburg, Illinois 60173
(800) LA–LECHE

La Leche League is a nonprofit, international organization with over 3,000 local support groups. It provides information and support to women who want to breast-feed their babies.

MOTHERS UNITED FOR MUTUAL SUPPORT (MUMS)
150 Custer Court
Green Bay, Wisconsin 54301
(414) 336–5333 fax (414) 339-0995

This organization is a parent–to–parent organization for parents or care providers of a child with *any* disability, disorder, chromosomal abnormality or health condition. It provides support to parents in the form of a networking system that matches them with other parents whose children have the same or similar condition.

MOTHERS WITHOUT CUSTODY (MWOC)
P.O. Box 36
Woodstock, Illinois 60098
(800) 457–MWOC

A national organization with local chapters offering support for women experiencing a custody battle, or who have lost custody of their children. A subscription to *"Mother–To–Mother"* is $25.00 per year.

NATIONAL BLACK WOMEN'S HEALTH PROJECT (NBWHP)
1237 Ralph David Abernathy Boulevard, SW
Atlanta, Georgia 30310
(404) 758–9590

NBWHP is a grassroots health advocacy organization, run by Black women for Black women. NBWHP has self–help support groups in 31 states, with over 100 self–help groups available. NBWHP is committed to defining, promoting and maintaining the physical, spiritual, mental and emotional well–being of Black women.

NATIONAL ORGANIZATION OF SINGLE MOTHERS, INC. (NOSM)
P.O. Box 68
Midland, North Carolina 28107
(704) 888–KIDS fax (704) 888-1752
NOSM is a national, non–profit organization dedicated to supporting single mothers through its local chapters and publication, SingleMOTHER.

THE NURTURING NETWORK
200 Clocktower Place, Suite 200A
P.O. Box 223099
Carmel, California 93922
(800) TNN–4MOM
Services of this organization include counseling, housing with member families, financial assistance, medical referrals, client employer mediation, mentor programs, adoption counseling, college transfers, parenting classes and child care referrals

PARENTS ANONYMOUS
675 West Foothill Boulevard, Suite 220
Claremont, California 91711
(909) 621–6184, fax (909) 625–6304
Local referrals to support groups for parents who have abused, or are afraid of abusing their babies and children.

PARENTS PLACE – THE PARENTING RESOURCE CENTER ON THE WEB
The Parents Place offers a wide range of information and articles for parents, and has a "Single Parenting Reading Room". They also offer a newsletter "Single Parenting in the Nineties."
Can be located by E–mail at: http://www.parentsplace

PARENTS WITHOUT PARTNERS INTERNATIONAL, INC. (PWP)
401 North Michigan Avenue
Chicago, Illinois 60611
(312) 644–6610
International organization with local chapters providing support for single–parents. Membership includes a subscription to *Single Parent Magazine*.

SINGLE MOTHERS BY CHOICE
P.O. Box 1642
Gracie Square Station
New York, New York 10028
(212) 988–0993
National organization with local chapters providing support and information to single women who have chosen or who are considering single–motherhood.

SOLO – A Guide for the Single Parent
A bi–monthly newsletter, offering support, information, and discussions concerning a variety of important issues related to single–parenting. Subscriptions cost $18.00 per year.
(800) 477–5877

THE STEPFAMILY ASSOCIATION OF AMERICA (SAA)
215 Centennial Mall South, Suite 212
Lincoln, Nebraska 68508–1834
(800) 735–0329 or (402) 477–7837 fax (402) 477–8317
National association with local chapters providing education and support to help step families succeed. Offers a quarterly publication: STEPFAMILIES.

CRISIS PREGNANCY CENTERS

CARENET
109 Carpenter Drive, Suite 100
Sterling, Virginia 20164
(703) 478–5661 fax (703) 478–5668
CareNet trains pregnancy care center workers and other individuals to participate in a network of practical care for women in unplanned pregnancies. Though this organization is Christian in its approach, it helps all women without regard to their religious affiliation. The network offers free pregnancy tests; birth, abstinence and post–abortion counseling; housing; parenting classes; and help with financial, medical, and material needs, including free maternity clothes and baby furniture

PLANNED PARENTHOOD FEDERATION OF AMERICA
810 7th Avenue
New York, New York 10019
(800) 230–PLAN (212) 541–7800
Local clinics offer counseling and referrals to services in your community. Many local clinics offer prenatal care. Look in your phone book for a clinic near you.

Note: For additional referrals, look in your phone book under Abortion Alternatives, Pregnancy Counseling, or Social and Human Services.

LOW–INCOME FAMILY SERVICES

ACORN
(202) 547-9292
Can assist women with low-to-moderate income in applying for, and getting, a loan to purchase a home.

THE FEDERAL INFORMATION CENTER
(800) 688–9889
can provide telephone numbers for information of all federal programs which may be available to you if you qualify.

HEAD START
Head Start has over 1,300 centers nationwide which offer education and support services for parents, including day care and educational programs for infants from low– income families. Call your local public school or Department of Social Services, or look in your phone book under "Head Start Centers."

HILL BURTON HOTLINE
(800) 638–0742
Provides information and referrals to local free hospital and medical care for low–income women and their children.

UNITED WAY
Provides referrals to a variety of local support services. Look in your white pages for the number of your local office.

WELFARE WARRIORS
2711 W. Michigan
Milwaukee, Wisconsin 53208
(414) 342–6662 – help line for low–income women) (414) 342–MOMS
A grass roots organization which provides information on government aid programs, education and job training, among other issues relevant to low–income mothers. Offers subscription to *Welfare Mothers Voice.*

YWCA
(212) 614–2700 to request a Worldwide directory or for a referral to a Y near you. Each Y offers its own curriculum to women in the community. Services include prenatal classes, support groups, career counseling, help for victims of abuse, among other opportunities to associate with other mothers

Additional resources include: WOMEN, INFANTS AND CHILDREN (WIC), food stamps, AID TO FAMILIES WITH DEPENDENT CHILDREN (AFDC), and Job Training (JOBS). Look in the government pages of your phone book for government aid services.

LEGAL SERVICES

ACADEMY OF FAMILY MEDIATORS
(617) 674-2663 fax (617) 674-2690
can provide a list of mediators in your state

ADMINISTRATION FOR CHILDREN AND FAMILIES
Office of Child Support Enforcement
Department of Health & Human Services
378 L'Enfant Promenade SW
Washington, DC 20447
(202) 401–9383
Offers information on how to establish paternity, collect child support, etc.

THE ASSOCIATION FOR CHILDREN FOR ENFORCEMENT OF SUP-PORT, INC. (ACES)
2260 Upton Avenue
Toledo, Ohio 43606
(800) 537–7072 – Hot Line
(419) 472–0047 fax (419) 472–6295
ACES is dedicated to assisting disadvantaged children affected by parents who fail to meet the legal and moral child support and/or visitation obligations. ACES offers educational programs, monthly chapter meetings, etc.

CHILDREN'S RIGHTS COUNCIL
220 I Street NE, #140
Washington, DC 20002
(800) 787-4KIDS (202) 547–6227 fax (202) 546-4272
CRC is a national non-profit organization. It provides referrals to mediators and local organizations in your area regarding visitation and chilc custody.

NOW LEGAL DEFENSE AND EDUCATION FUND
99 Hudson Street
New York, New York 10013
(212) 925–6635
Offers information kits ($5.00) on pregnancy discrimination issues, divorce, child support, custody.

Note: For a referral to a local attorney, call your local bar association, woman's bar association, or Legal Aid Society

MENTAL HEALTH/COUNSELING SERVICES

AMERICAN ACADEMY OF CHILD AND ADOLESCENT PSYCHIATRY
3615 Wisconsin Avenue NW
Washington, DC 20016
(202) 966–7300

AMERICAN ASSOCIATION OF PASTORAL COUNSELORS
9504A Lee Highway
Fairfax, Virginia 22031
(703) 385–6967
Provides local referrals

DEPRESSION AFTER DELIVERY
P.O. Box 1282
Morrisville, Pennsylvania 19067
(800) 944–4773 – (215) 295–3994
Provides a list of support groups and telephone contacts for mothers suffering from postpartum depression.

NATIONAL MENTAL HEALTH ASSOCIATION
1021 Prince Street
Alexandra, Virginia 22314
(703) 684–7722
Provides referrals to local therapy/counseling providers

NATIONAL CLEARINGHOUSE FAMILY SUPPORT/CHILDREN'S MENTAL HEALTH
(800) 628–1696
Referrals to local family clinics, support groups, counselors and therapists

NATIONAL GRIEF RECOVERY
(800) 445–4808
Helps those suffering from the loss of a loved one.

PHYSICAL HEALTH SERVICES

AMERICAN ACADEMY OF PEDIATRICS, PEDIATRICIAN REFERRAL
141 Northwest Point Boulevard
Elk Grove, Illinois 60009–0927
(847) 228-5005

THE AMERICAN COLLEGE OF OBSTETRICIANS AND GYNECOLO-GISTS
409 12th Street, S.W.
Washington, DC 20024–2188
(202) 484–3321
Provides information on pregnancy and women's health.

CESAREAN/SUPPORT, EDUCATION AND CONCERN
22 Forest Road, Framingham, MA 01701
(508) 877–8266

THE NATIONAL MATERNAL AND CHILD HEALTH CLEARING-HOUSE/CIRCLE SOLUTIONS
(703) 821–8955
provides referrals to local health care providers.

DONOR INSEMINATION RESOURCES

BIOGENETICS
(800) 637-7776

CALIFORNIA CRYOBANK
(800) 231–3373

ZYGEN LABORATORY
(800) 255–7242

XYTEX CORPORATION
(800) 277–3210

PACES CRYOBANK AND INFERTILITY SERVICES
(404) 252–7049

WORK

BUSINESS AND PROFESSIONAL WOMEN'S FOUNDATION (BWP)
(202) 293–1100
BWP promotes "equity and economic self–sufficiency for working women through educational programs, research, community awareness, and personal development."

9 TO 5
1430 W. Peachtree Street, #600
Atlanta, Georgie 30309
(800) 522-0925
9 To 5 is a national working woman's advocacy group.

COALITION OF LABOR UNION WOMEN
1126 16th Street NW, Washington, DC 20036
(202) 296–1200 x210
Offers referrals to union help in your area

DEPARTMENT OF LABOR
Women's Bureau Clearinghouse
200 Constitution Avenue NW, Washington, DC 20210
(800) 827–5335
Provides information on pregnancy discrimination, family medical leave, and sexual harassment.

MOTHERS' HOME BUSINESS NETWORK
P.O. Box 423, East Meadow, New York 11554
(516) 997–7394
Provides information to women to explore options to work from home. A $35.00 membership includes a subscription to *Homeworking Mothers* newsletter.

NATIONAL ASSOCIATION FOR FEMALE EXECUTIVES (NAFE)
(800) 927–6233
This group offers help to women interested in networking and furthering her career. They offer a resume database, skill–building seminars and satellite conferences.

EDUCATION/EMPLOYMENT AND TRAINING RESOURCES

GED HOTLINE
(800) 626–9433

CLEARINGHOUSE ON ADULT CAREER AND VOCATIONAL EDUCA-TION
(800) 848–4815

CHILDBIRTH CLASSES

ASPO – LAMAZE
1200 19th Street NW, Suite 300, Washington, DC 20036
(800) 368–4404

THE BRADLEY METHOD
(800) 4–A–BIRTH

THE GRANT DICK–READ ASSOCIATION
(The Gamper Method)
(312) 248–8100

CRISIS HOTLINES – MISCELLANEOUS

AL–ANON FAMILY GROUP HEADQUARTERS
(800) 356–9996

ALCOHOLICS ANONYMOUS
468 Park Avenue South
New York, New York
For a local number, look in your local directory

BOYS TOWN CHILD ABUSE HOTLINE
(800) 448–3000

CHILDHELP USA CHILD ABUSE HOTLINE
(800) 422–4453

CHILDREN'S RIGHTS OF AMERICA
(800) 442–4673

HIV/AIDS Treatment Information Services
(800) 448–0440

NATIONAL AIDS HOTLINE
(800) 342–2437

NATIONAL AIDS INFORMATION CLEARINGHOUSE
(800) 458–5231

NATIONAL CENTER FOR MISSING AND EXPLOITED CHILDREN
(800) 843–5678

NATIONAL COUNCIL ON CHILD ABUSE AND FAMILY VIOLENCE
(800) 222–2000

NATIONAL DRUG HOTLINE
(800) 662–4357
treatment and referrals

NATIONAL HELPLINE FOR SUBSTANCE ABUSE
(800) 262-2463

NATIONAL RUNAWAY SWITCHBOARD
(800) 621–4000

NATIONAL RESOURCE CENTER FOR CHILD ABUSE AND NE-GLECT
(800) 227–5242

CHILD CARE

CHILD CARE AWARE
2116 Campus Drive SE
Rochester, MN 55904
(800) 424–2246
(507) 287–2220 fax (507) 287–2411
The mission of Child Care Aware is to improve the quality of child care in America by supporting professional development and training programs, and by educating parents to recognize and choose good child care. The toll–free national information line links parents with child care resources and referral agencies in their own communities.

DEPARTMENT OF LABOR
Work and Family Clearinghouse
(800) 827–5335
Provides information to employers about day care centers, flexible–leave policies

NATIONAL WORK AND FAMILY ALLIANCE
(415) 931–7640
Provides information on child care and solutions for working parents

ADVOCACY – POLITICAL

THE LEAGUE OF WOMEN'S VOTERS
1730 M Street NW
Washington, DC 20036
(202) 429-1965
The League is a national non–profit, non–partisan organization dedicated to help promote citizens in government. They educate people through public forums on the pros and cons of issues, and run voter registration drives.

RECOMMENDED READING

SINGLE PREGNANCIES – SINGLE PARENTING

Single Mothers by Choice: A Guidebook For Single Women Who Are Considering or Have Chosen Motherhood by Jane Mattes (Random House/Times Books)

Two Of Us Make A World: The Single Mother's Guide to Pregnancy, Childbirth, and the First Year by Prudence and Sherill Tippins (An Owl Book/Henry Holt and Company)

Joy of Single Mothering: Reassuring Answers to Your Most Challenging Concerns by Andrea Engber (Bob Adams)

Solo Parenting – Your Essential Guide: How to Find the Balance Between Parenthood and Personhood by Kathleen McCoy (A Plume Book/New American Library)

The Single Mother's Book by Joan Anderson (Peachtree Publishers)

PREGNANCY AND PARENTING ISSUES – GENERAL/ SPECIAL INTEREST

The Hite Report on the Family: Growing up Under Patriarchy, by Shere Hite (Grove Press) – includes a section on single–parent families.

Your Baby & Child – From Birth to Age Five, by Penelope Leach (Alfred A. Knopf)

What to Expect When You're Expecting, by Arlene Eisenberg, Heidi E. Murkoff, and Sandee E. Hathaway, B.S.N. (Workman Publishing)

Complete Pregnancy & Baby Book, by Vicki Lansky & Consumer Guide Editors (Publications International)

The Secret Life of the Unborn Child, by Thomas Verny, M.D., with John Kelly (A Dell Trade Paperback)

The Baby Book: Everything You Need to Know About Your Baby from Birth to Age Two, by William Sears and Martha Sears (Little Brown and Company)

Not in Front of the Children, by Lawrence Balter and Peggy Donahue (Viking Penguin)

The Six Stages of Parenthood, by Ellen Galinsky (Addison–Wesley Publishing)

In Vitro Fertilization – The A.R.T.* of Making Babies/Revised Edition, by Geoffrey Sher, M.D., Virginia Marriage Davis, R.N., M.N., and Jean Stoess, M.A., Facts On File/An Infobase Holdings Company

DISCIPLINE AND DEVELOPMENT

Who's in Control? Dr. Balter's Guide to Discipline Without Combat, by Lawrence Balter with Anita Shreve (Poseidon Press)

Your Child's Emotional and Behavioral Development, The Essential Reference, by T. Berry Brazelton (Addison–Wesley Publishing)

Discipline That Works: Promoting Self–Discipline in Children at Home and at School, by Gordon Thomas (N.A.L. Dutton)

HEALTH ISSUES

What to Eat When You're Expecting, by Arlene Eisenberg, Heidi E. Murkoff, and Sandee E. Hathaway, B.S.N. (Workman Publishing)

How To Raise a Healthy Child...In Spite of Your Doctor, by Robert S. Mendelsohn, M.D. (Ballantine Books)

The Immunization Decision – A Guide for Parents, by Randall Neustaedter (North Atlantic Books)

Vaccination and Immunisation: Dangers, Delusions and Alternatives (What Every Parent Should Know), by Leon Chaitow (The C.W. Daniel Company Ltd)

DIVORCE ISSUES

Helping Your Child Through Your Divorce, by Florence Bienenfeld, Ph.D. (Hunter House)

Divorce and Child Custody – Your Options and Legal Rights, by Deanna Peters and Richard L. Strohm (Career Press)

You're Entitled, by Sidney M . D'Angelis (Contemporary Books)

WORKING MOTHERS

Everything a Working Mother Needs to Know About Pregnancy Rights, Maternity Leave, and Making Her Career Work for Her, by Anne C. Weisberg and Carol A. Buckler (Main Street Books, Doubleday)

From Paycheck to Power: The Working Woman's Guide to Reducing Debt, Building Assets and Getting What You Want Out of Life, by Anne Owings Wilson and Linda Bessette (August House)

Working Mothers, by Jean Curtis (Doubleday)

TIME MANAGEMENT

Organize Your Family: Simple Routines for You and Your Kids, by Ronnie Eisenberg (Hyperion)

MONEY MATTERS

The Budget Kit: The Common Cent$ Money Management Workbook, by Judy Lawrence (Dearborn Financial Publishing)

Great Buys for Kids: How to Save Money on Everything for Children and Teens, by Sue Goldstein (Viking Penguin)

The Dollars and Sense Guide to Divorce: The Financial Guide for Women, by Judith Briles (Ballantine)

Money Smart: Secrets Women Need to Know About Money, by Esther M. Berger, CFP, with Connie Church Hasbun (Simon & Schuster)

BOOKS FOR CHILDREN

Tell Me No Lies, by Hila Colman (Crown Publishers)

It's Not the End of the World, by Judy Blume (Bradbury Press)

My Kind of Family: A Book for Kids in Single–Parent Homes (Waterfront Books)

The Boys' and Girls' Book About One Parent Families (Bantam Books)

Do I Have A Daddy? (Yo tengo papa?) (Morning Glory Press)

How It Feels When Parents Divorce (Alfred A. Knopf)

How It Feels to Be Adopted (Alfred A. Knopf)

How It Feels When a Parent Dies (Alfred A. Knopf)

Heather Has Two Mommies (Ayson Publications)

DATING AND THE SINGLE MOTHER

Love Me, Love My Kids, A Guide for the New Partner, by Peter Rowlands (Continuum)

CHILD CARE

The Complete Guide to Choosing Child Care, by Judith Berezin (Random House)

BIBLIOGRAPHY

A Doctor Discusses Pregnancy; by William G. Birch, M.D., L.L.D., (Hon); Budlong Press Company

Complete Pregnancy & Baby Book; by Vicki Lansky & Consumer Guide Editors; Publications International, Ltd.

How to Change Your Life, Dr. Ernest Holmes; Science of Mind Communications

The Hite Report on the Family: Growing up Under Patriarchy; by Shere Hite   Grove Press

Love is Letting Go of Fear; Gerald G. Jampolsky, M.D.; Bantam Books

Love Me, Love My Kids, A Guide for the New Partner; by Peter Rowlands; Continuum

The Mommy Guide; by Susan Bernard; Contemporary Books

The Secret Life of the Unborn Child; by Thomas Verny, M.D., with John Kelly; A Dell Trade Paperback

The Single Mother's Book; by Joan Anderson; Peachtree Publishers

Student Handbook, College and University Edition, Volume Four, (Development, p: 446–454); Southwestern

The Well Baby Book; by Mike Samuels, M.D., and Nancy Samuels; Simon and Schuster

What To Expect When You're Expecting; by Arlene Eisenberg, Heidi E. Murkoff, and Sandee E. Hathaway, B.S.N.; Workman Publishing

What To Expect The First Year; by Arlene Eisenberg, Heidi E. Murkoff, and Sandee E. Hathaway, B.S.N.; Workman Publishing

Your Baby & Child – From Birth to Age Five/New Edition; by Penelope Leach; Alfred A. Knopf

Commentary; "The National Prospect: A Symposium"; November, 1995; p:23–39; by William F. Buckley

Education Digest; "Family Patterns Today"; February, 1995; p:47–49; by Peter L. Benson

Essence; "Doing it Solo"; October, 1995; p:122–126; by Joy Duckett Cain

Futurist; "Reversing Fatherlessness–Fatherless America – Confronting Our Most Urgent Social Problem" (abstract); September, 1995; p:61–62; by David Blankenhorn

Growing Up Drug Free – A Parent's Guide To Prevention; 1996; U.S. Department of Education, Washington, DC

Index of Leading Cultural Indicators; Volume I, 1993; William J. Bennett

Nation; "A Program to Help Working Parents"; May, 1995; p:592–595; by Barbara R. Bergman and Heidi I. Hartman

New York Times; "Welfare is No Incentive"; July, 1994 (abstract); p:27

Parenting Pages – California Consortium to Prevent Child Abuse; "Parents Are Teachers Too"; April, 1995; p:2–3; by Jean C. Monroe

Parenting Pages – California Consortium to Prevent Child Abuse; "Styles of Family Communication"; April, 1995; p:5; by the Family & Relationship Center

Parenting Pages – California Consortium to Prevent Child Abuse; "Discipline is Not a Dirty Word"; April, 1995; p:1; by Jennifer Birkmayter

Time; "Faith & Healing'" June, 1996; by Caludia Wallis

Time; "The Myth About Welfare Moms"; July, 1995; p:21; by Michael Kramer

Total Health; "Exercise During Pregnancy"; December, 1995; p:11; by Robert Smith

USA Today; "Out–of–Wedlock Childbirth Rising"; November, 1995; p:2; by Mark Potok

US News & World Report; "One Child in Four is in a Single–Parent Home"; p:6; anonymous

Vogue; "Menace to Society"; December, 1994; p:88–92; by Stephanie Coontz

Women's Sports & Fitness; "Hoop Reality"; May, 1995; p:30–32; anonymous

Working Mothers: by Jean Curtis (Doubleday & Company)

ParentsPlace.com/SPN Home Page;"Identifying Depression In Children"; by Penny E. Stone

ParentsPlace.com/SPN Home Page; "Developing A Healthy Self–Esteem In Your Child" (abstract); from Single Parenting in the Nineties

INDEX

SINGLE PREGNANCY – SINGLE PARENTING
Empowering the Single Parent, By Keri Bowers

To order by mail, just call toll–free 1-888-BABY AND ME (222-9263) or send your order to:

Park Alexander Press
P.O. Box 23785
Pleasant Hill, CA 94523

	Price:	U.S.	Canada
___ Copies of SINGLE PREGNANCY – SINGLE PARENTING		$12.95	$16.95
___ Copies of MEDITATION AND YOUR UNBORN CHILD(Cassette)		$10.00	$14.00
___ Copies of MOTHER'S MEDITATION (Cassette)		$10.00	$14.00

Subtotal $ _____

Less 20% for 3 or more books ordered $ _____

*Postage and handling $ _____

Sales Tax (CA, NJ, NY, PA) $ _____

Total Amount Due $ _____

Payable in U.S. Funds (No cash orders accepted)
* Postage & handling $3.10 for one book, $.75 cents for each additional book up to a maximum of $6.00.

Enclosed is my   [   ] check   [   ] money order
Please charge my   [   ] Visa   [   ] MasterCard   [   ]American Express

Card#_____ Expiration date_____

*Signature as on charge card*_____

Name_____

Address_____

City_____State_____Zip_____

Please allow 3–6 weeks for delivery. Prices subject to change without notice.